All about Your Cat's Health

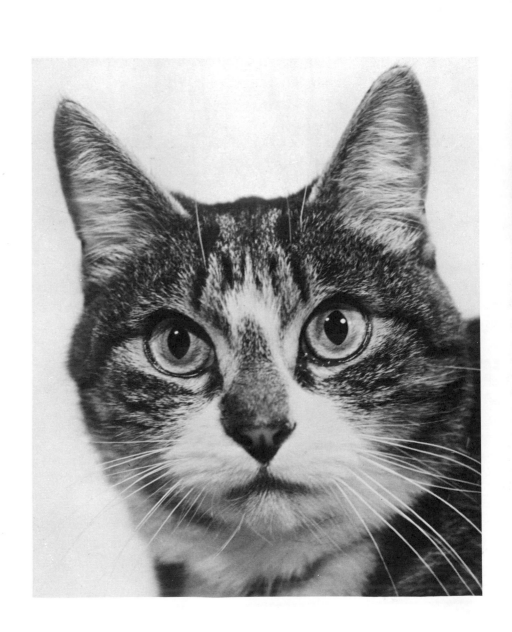

All about
Your Cat's Health

GEOFFREY WEST M.R.C.V.S.

PELHAM BOOKS

First published in Great Britain by
Pelham Books Ltd
44 Bedford Square
London WC1B 3DU
1980

West, Geoffrey Philip
   All about your cats' health.
   1. Cats — Diseases
   I. Title
   636.8'08'96   SF985

ISBN 0 7207 1277 7

Set, printed and bound in Singapore

Contents

List of Illustrations

Acknowledgements

ILLUSTRATION ACKNOWLEDGEMENTS

The author and publishers would like to thank the following for permission to use copyright material:
Agricultural Research Council (28)
Animal Virus Research Institute, Pirbright (51)
Trustees of the British Museum (1, 2, 3)
Mrs Irene Campbell (K)
Carnation Company, U.S.A. (20, 44)
R.E. Chaplin (10)
Miss Dawn Critchley (A)
Dorset News (38)
S.W. Douglas, M.A., M.R.C.V.S., D.V.R., Dept of Clinical Veterinary Studies, University of Cambridge (39, 46, 47)
Ethicon Ltd (B, 19, G, 35, 49, L, P)
Marc Henrie and Pedigree Petfoods (frontispiece, 13, 21, 23, 24, 25, F, 32, 33, 34, 35, I, J, 50, M, N)
Dr C.J. La Touche and the University of London (26, 27, 31)
Mr and Mrs Mc Kenzie (16)
Milk Marketing Board (29)
Press Association (8, 11)
Mrs Janet Romer (9,0)
Royal Veterinary College (36, 37, 41)
Dr G. Schneck, M.R.C.V.S., Graz, Austria (30, 42, 43, 45, 48)
John Smith Baxter, B.V.M.S., M.R.C.V.S., (18)
World Health Organisation (52)

Photographs 5, 6, 7, C, 14, 15, 18, D, E, 22, and 53 are copyright of the author, Geoffrey West, M.R.C.V.S.

TEXT ACKNOWLEDGEMENTS

The author and publishers are grateful to the following for permission to reproduce copyright material: Thames and Hudson Ltd. for the quote from *Dogs, Cats and People* by Norman Comben; Cambridge University Press for the extract from *The Cat in Ancient Egypt* by N. and B. Langton; A.P. Watt Ltd. for the extract from *C is for Cat* by Dr Frank Manolson (1965 edition); Macmillan Publishers Ltd. for the extract from *The Macmillan Treasury of Relevant Quotations* by Edward F. Murphy; Clarke, Irwin Co. Ltd., Toronto, for the extract from *The Table Talk of Samuel Marchbanks* by Robertson Davies.

I should like to acknowledge my indebtedness to all those veterinary surgeons whose names are given in the references or in the text. My thanks are also offered to Mr Edward Boden, Editor of the *Veterinary Record,* for permission to make abstracts from papers or letters; to Miss B. Horder, Librarian at the Royal College of Veterinary Surgeons, and her staff; and to Mr A.T.B. Edney, past President, British Small Animal Veterinary Association, for kindly reading with a critical eye chapters 2 to 22. To all those who have helped with illustrations I am most grateful; particularly so to Professor A.O. Betts, Principal of the Royal Veterinary College, University of London; Mr R. Churchill Frost, University of London; to Pedigree Petfoods Education Centre; Ethicon Ltd. and Carnation Company U.S.A.

Preface

This is not just another cat book. It is different. There are several which offer good advice on first-aid; and some which mention briefly a few illnesses. It seemed to the author that cat owners might prefer something in greater depth, which would offer explanations, dilate a little on cause and effect, and be a source of information on feline ills not available hitherto in a book with this readership in mind.

Not *all* of the conditions described are common (indeed some are rare), but it is felt that an owner encountering a less familiar one will be glad of information about it. Busy veterinary surgeons, with a waiting-room full of clients and patients, do not always have as much time as they would like for explanations. Moreover, they sometimes use technical terms, many of which may be meaningless to the cat's owner. Accordingly, a glossary has been provided.

A unique feature of this book is the extensive use of case histories, both to amplify and enliven the text. Some are based on the author's own experience in practice; others have been abstracted (and shorn of technical jargon) from the veterinary literature of several countries.

An index will help the reader; but so, it is hoped, will the grouping of topics under appropriate chapter headings; e.g. 'Accidents and Other Emergencies', 'The Itchy Cat', 'The Thirsty Cat', etc.

Causes, symptoms, first-aid or prevention are given, as appropriate; with emphasis on avoidance of trouble, so far as this is possible. There is a whole chapter devoted to the subject of rabies. To put the whole into perspective, there is the opening chapter 'The Cat in Society'.

Finally, it should be stated that this is not intended as a 'do-it-yourself' book (apart from first-aid). On the contrary, the need for professional diagnosis and treatment is stressed throughout.

1 The Cat in Society

Before discussing feline health, illnesses, accidents, preventive measures and first-aid, with which this book is mainly concerned, a brief look at the cat's place in society seems highly relevant. Social attitudes towards cats, ever since their domestication, must always have affected their health and well-being.

Domestication

When and where cats were first domesticated, history does not relate, but it is known that there were tame cats in Egypt about 3,500 years before Christ. Herodotus, that widely travelled Greek historian who was born in 484 B.C., referred to the strangely exaggerated regard for the cat felt by the dwellers on the Nile. He noted that when a cat died, Egyptians shaved off their eyebrows as a sign of mourning.

Fig 1
A bronze figure of a cat with gold earrings, popular in ancient Egypt.

Fig 2
The mummy of an Egyptian cat. Cats were sacred to the goddess Bastet, whose popularity as a protective deity increased after 600 B.C. This mummy dates from the Roman Period, after 30 B.C.

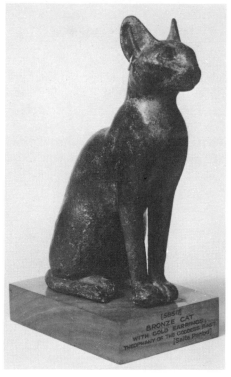
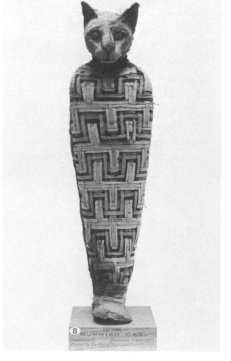

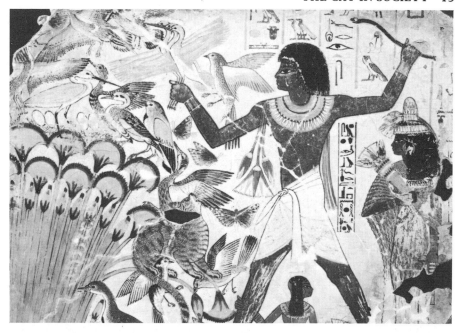

Fig 3
A specially trained
hunting cat, taking a
bird knocked down by
a noble's throw-stick,
as depicted in an
ancient papyrus.

Whereas dogs played only a very minor role in religious observances —
turning prayer-wheels in Tibet — cats were sacred animals not only in ancient
Egypt but also in the New World to the Aztecs and pre-Incan people.

In ancient Egypt the cat goddess was worshipped as a goddess of light, love,
and hunting, and a surviving papyrus refers to a privilege conferred on the
feeders of the sacred cats.

'The number of cat figures that have survived is the best possible evidence
of the popularity of Bastet as the cat goddess', commented the Langtons;[1] and
they range from life-size to tiny pieces 'almost too small for carving, and of
every material from gold to mud'. Examples of cat figures, and also of cat
mummies, can be seen in the British Museum. Charles Darwin accepted
another expert's opinion that these Egyptian cat mummies were of three
distinct species: *Felis caligulata, F. bybastes,* and *F. chaus,* and his view was
that our domestic cats are descendants of several species, including these. *F.
lybica* of North Africa, *F. caffra* of South Africa, and four Indian species, all
cross readily with domestic cats, as does *F. sylvestris,* the wild cat of Scotland.

The ancient Egyptians' reverence for the cat was turned to their disadvan-
tage by King Cambyses (d. 522 B.C.), whose success in conquering Egypt has
been attributed in part to his soldiers driving cats in front of them, so that the
Egyptian archers dared not shoot.

Apart from sacred cats and pet cats, others rendered great service by killing
rats and so protecting Egypt's granaries. Egyptian nobles hunted with trained
cats, which were released to put up ducks in the marshes, and to retrieve
waterfowl knocked down by their masters' throwsticks.

In China and Japan, as well as in ancient Greece and Rome, cats obtained protection and friendship from human beings. Gregory I, the great Pope from 590-604, is said to have had a pet cat, and many nunneries had cats as inmates during the Middle Ages. A canon, enacted in 1127, forbade any abbess or nun to wear more costly fur than that of a cat.

In Britain, Dr St George Mivat F.R.S. wrote: 'When Julius Caesar landed here, our forests were plentifully supplied with cats, while probably not a single mouser existed in any town or village.' In the thirteenth century cats were hunted in the royal forests, and the Abbot of Peterborough was among those who received a charter from King Richard II granting permission to hunt the cat. The Middle Ages were bad times for cats, and much cruelty was perpetrated on them. Superstition played a big part in this, and when witches were burned at the stake, their cats shared the same fate. However, towards the end of this period several European countries enacted laws which imposed a heavy fine on cat-killers.

It seems that the Great Plague of 1664-65 helped to boost the popularity of cats among Londoners, who had good reason to appreciate cats' rat-killing ability, still esteemed today by farmers, grain merchants, government departments and householders.

'The tendency to catch rats rather than mice is known to be inherited,' wrote Charles Darwin, who stated that cats vary in their choice of prey; some preferring rats, some mice, some birds, others hares or rabbits; with marsh-frequenting cats 'bringing home almost nightly woodcock and snipe'. A century or two ago, it seems, domestic cats with a liking for hunting were still regarded in hamlets and villages as useful providers of food. Edith Carrington, a nineteenth-century writer on cats, referred to the habit of some of them of offering prey to human beings as 'a token of regard', and instanced

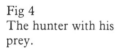

Fig 4
The hunter with his prey.

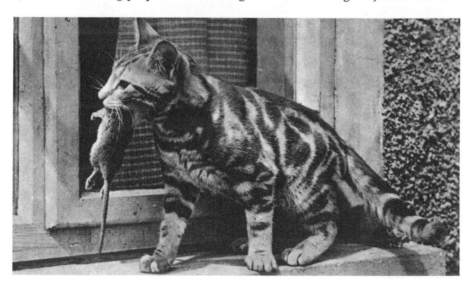

her own cat's 'six neatly arranged corpses of mouse, sparrow, butterfly and three cockroaches'.

Cats are often accused of being cruel; but are they? The mother cat brings back, let us say, a mouse which has been nipped to make difficult its escape, and lets her kittens kill it. She teaches them how to do it. They practise, increasing the accuracy of their pounce; and when they grow older and hunt for themselves they continue to practise — which is not to say that they do not also enjoy it. Who knows?

Robert Southey wrote of cats: 'He who supposes that animals have not their different dispositions as well as man, knows very little of animal nature', and this is undoubtedly true. Some cats are affectionate and, at times, seem full of *joie de vivre*. Others tend to hold themselves aloof; their habitual appearance suggests apathy or boredom; they are undemonstrative, and do not jump on to people's laps and purr. 'God made the cat in order that man might have the pleasure of caressing the tiger', wrote Fernand Méry; and indeed something of the tiger lurks in every cat.

Charles Baudelaire wrote: 'A cat is beautiful; it suggests ideas of luxury, cleanliness, and voluptuous pleasures.' Robertson Davies was less flattering: 'Cats are disdainful of everything but their own immediate interests, and they contrive to be so suave and delightful about it that they receive the apotheosis of a National Week.' Edith Carrington commented: 'There is hardly any cat which will not rise from her seat to meet the blandishments of a guest half way, with a subtle blending of dignity and humility — a dash of effusiveness subdued by self-respect.'

Cats and Cars

To say that cats like cars is not strictly true. They like *parked* cars. The tyres have interesting smells, and the shady underside of an automobile offers excellent tactical possibilities. In winter, too, the warm bonnet of a recently used car has distinct amenity value. Except to the rare feline eccentric, however, a moving car is an abomination. Most people know this and do not subject their cats to enforced motoring unless they have borrowed or possess a carrying cage or basket designed expressly for this purpose and in a good state of repair. Even then, if they are wise, on some pretext or other they obtain the use of someone else's car.

The Lancet, many years ago, contained an engaging account of a physiologist who was cast for the role of Someone Else. He had spent a rather trying social weekend at a house

> where cats in quantity were kept for decorative purposes. The doyen of the establishment, a large and cynical ginger tom, had taken to looking upon the house as a sort of second-rate hotel serving indifferent meals. He lived now in the rafters of a disused outhouse, and visited the house

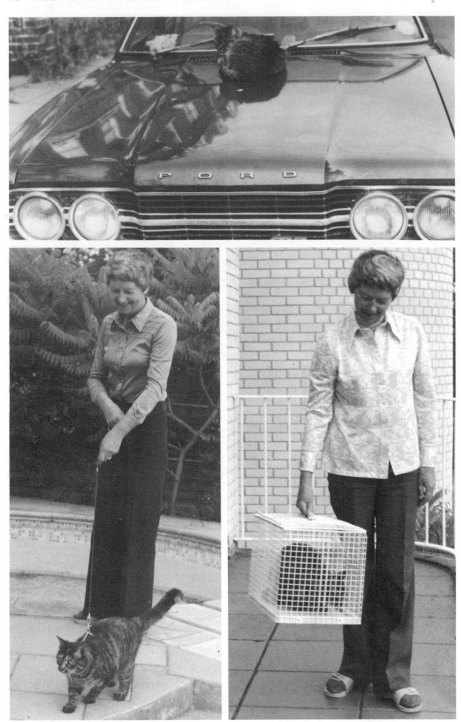

Fig 5
A warm car bonnet for comfort.
Fig 6
Frisky has been familiarised with a carrying cage – so much more satisfactory than a cat basket, as the animal can see all round, and cleaning is easy.
Fig 7
Accustoming a cat to collar and lead from an early age can obviate problems in later life. Mrs J.C. Scriven with Frisky.

at rare intervals speaking to no one. It was felt by my hosts that the cat was not pulling its weight, and the Physiologist — accepted as an animal fancier in view of his deep knowledge of the internal workings of the Wistar rat — was deputed to catch the cat and take him hence.

The commission was recklessly accepted, and our hero — armed with the strength of his personality and a hat-box — approached his quarry during its siesta by means of a long ladder. The cat observed the operation dreamily, and — tired by the exertions of the night — offered a purely formal protest which caused the Physiologist, however, to fall down four rungs and nearly lost him the sight of an eye. After which, the cat suffered itself to be placed in the hat-box. This was securely tied with string and placed on the back seat of the car.

By the first traffic lights it became evident that the feline passenger was taking itself to task for allowing itself to be imposed upon. A hat-box was one thing, a moving car quite another. At the second traffic lights the Physiologist looked round at the sound of a sinister tearing noise and observed a yellow eye regarding him savagely through a jagged hole in the hat-box. Before any steps could be taken, the animal had become fully abreast of the situation and emerged as if propelled by a blasting charge. The car seemed to be full of cats which flashed past, upsetting ashtrays, disrupting upholstery and dismantling armrests. Finally, as the Physiologist put it, one of the multitude landed squarely on the top of his head and shot out of the driver's window.

It took some little time to staunch the flow of blood from his shredded scalp, but when the Physiologist eventually arrived back at his hosts' house the cat was once more in residence in the outhouse, enjoying a well-earned nap.

Cats as Life-savers and Travellers

There are several stories of cats saving human lives through giving warning of impending disasters, but the one I like best was related by the late Dr Frank Manolson M.R.C.V.S.,[2] and concerned a Persian which had, for fifteen years, shown utter disdain for an American family. Then, one night, he jumped on to the bed and awoke his sleeping 'owners' by patting their faces with his paws and pulling at the bedclothes. So unusual was this that the couple went downstairs and looked around the house. What they found was that coal stored in the basement was smouldering, 'and in minutes would have got beyond control'. They made a fuss of the cat, but next day he reverted to his former disdainful aloofness.

Cats were carried into battle as mascots by the Ancient Egyptians, and they have been carried into battle in modern times by ships of the Royal Navy. I am indebted to a former Bishop of St Helena, the Right Reverend Harold

Beardmore, O.B.E., for the mention of a cat called Fishcakes, mascot of H.M.S. *Hood*. This animal was joined by the future Bishop's bull-terrier, Bill. When, on appointment as chaplain to the Flagship, Bill's owner descended *Hood*'s gangway for the last time, the quartermaster said: 'We're very sorry you're leaving us, sir, and especially Bill, our mascot. Now I suppose our luck will change, and we'll have to rely on Fishcakes.' A few months later came the tragic loss of H.M.S. *Hood*, from which there were but three survivors. For the first time in her life, Fishcakes had remained in a Fleet oiler which had come alongside to refuel the ship, and had not sailed in H.M.S. *Hood*.

For centuries there have been sea-going ship's cats. A modern liner's cat is referred to in chapter 23. Many yachtsmen have taken their cats along with them, and I recall reading of the dilemma of one crew who had left their Siamese ashore but had to move the boat to a different part of the harbour before the animal's return. The next they saw of it was swimming across the harbour to its floating home.

Many cats travel in ships and aircraft, either with their owners or otherwise. During a trans-Atlantic voyage in the liner *Queen Elizabeth II* I saw several cats housed in hygienic cages, with attendants on hand and owners free to visit.

Fig 8
A much travelled cat. Her box was found to be empty on arrival of a Pan Am Jumbo jet at Miami after a flight from Guam. She was not rescued until thirty-two days later, when – after a flight from San Francisco – baggage handlers found her in the hold, so weak that she could barely lift her head. Despite starvation, thirst, and the terror induced by noise and vibration, she is seen here, well on the way to recovery, in the arms of Julie Hyett, a quarantine station assistant at Heathrow.

Cats' Enemies

What of cats' enemies? Even today, human beings must be classed as cats' worst enemies. Tormenting children, sadistic youths, and a few ruthless gardeners (who set snares, or traps, or resort to airguns or shotguns) are among the offenders, as well as cat thieves, some of whom sell cats to disreputable laboratories. Greyhounds are notorious cat-killers and, of the wild animals, the fox has a similar reputation; though it must be added that while many cats are terrified of foxes, others are aggressive towards them, and a few are friendly.

Some of the nicest cats can be destructive in their own homes, to the extent that in their 'claw sharpening' they damage furniture, fabrics, and wallpaper. This topic is discussed in chapter 4. Nocturnal caterwauling is, from the human standpoint, one of the few other example of feline antisocial behaviour; so is the 'calling' of the queen (see chapter 20) which may disturb people.

Cats do not like noise either. 'I know one Siamese', wrote Dr Louis J. Camuti in *Feline Practice*, 'which hates the telephone. If she happens to be in the vicinity when it rings, she jumps up and knocks the receiver from its cradle.'

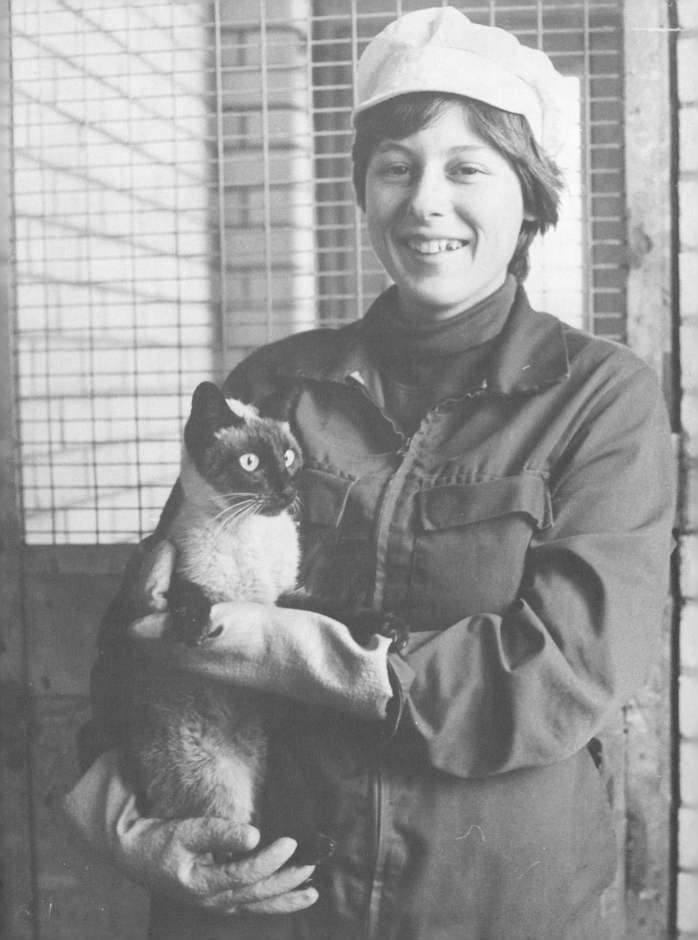

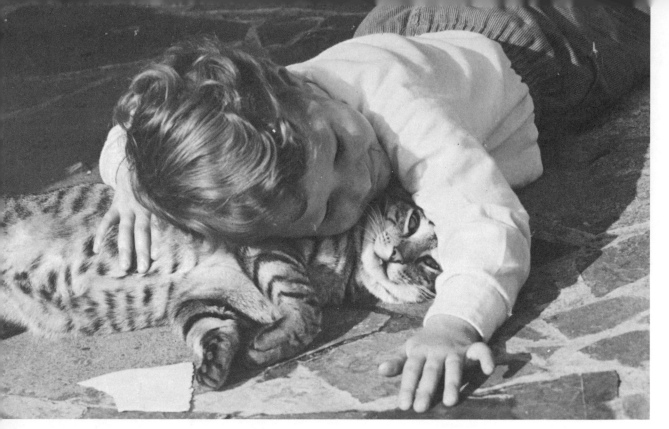

Fig 9
A picture of happiness,
but it is important that
children are
discouraged from
becoming boisterous
with cats.

Stray Cats

The stray cat problem is largely a man-made one. It can be reduced by the neutering of cats of both sexes, and by avoiding on-the-spur-of-the-moment purchase of kittens at Christmas and other times. As to reducing the existing number of strays, animal welfare societies (such as the Cats Protection League) and local authorities, often taking concerted action, can both help. Many semi-feral cats have to be 'put down' but some, even toms, can be 'rehabilitated' after neutering and, in due course, found homes.

Cat Mania

One can applaud, too, many private individuals who offer a home to a stray; but those who misguidedly take in all the stray cats they can collect are creating additional problems. Every practising veterinary surgeon has been into houses where there were far too many cats, including unneutered males, and the whole place reeked of the entire cat's urine.

Dr Denis Leigh, invited to present a paper at the 1966 annual congress of the British Small Animal Veterinary Association, referred to two old ladies whom he visited. Their homes

were remarkable. Flaps had been cut into all the doors so that the cats could pass freely all over the house, and the kitchen was devoted almost entirely to the cooking of fish. The toilet needs of the animals were provided for in every room. Both ladies had begun their 'cat mania' when over the age of sixty. The poor husbands were desperate.

In one case reported in a newspaper, a husband was stated to be living in a shed in the garden, having taken refuge from his home, which had become unbearable owing to the number of cats and the smell. His wife had given up her own bed to the cats.

Such extreme conditions are obviously to be deplored, and are far removed from responsible pet ownership; indeed, they may even impose stress on the feline inmates. Entire tom cats spray their urine indoors, as a result of stress, when their number is increased.

In contradistinction to this 'cat mania' is the companionship which a pet cat or two can provide. At another B.S.A.V.A. congress Dr R. Ryder, chief psychologist at an Oxford clinic, rejected the notion that human feelings towards animals were unnatural, sentimental, or pathetic. Pet animals, he maintained, were an excellent help in combating the stress of modern life; and pet-facilitated psychotherapy (P.F.P.) is well recognised in America.

Sometimes the cat is the object of human envy, and newspapers not infrequently contain reports of costly legal actions by the relatives of a deceased person over large sums of money left to support a pet cat. John Kerr, reporting from Milan in the *Daily Express,* told the story of a rich industrial-

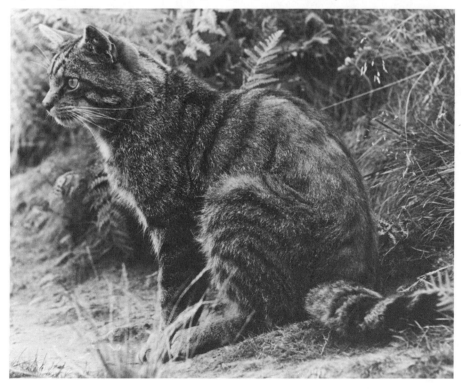

Fig 10
The wild cat of Scotland (*Felis sylvestris*), photographed by Raymond E. Chaplin, BSc., and looking very different from the snarling creature so often depicted. The tail is bushy and short, and the fur on the legs has thick, transverse stripes.

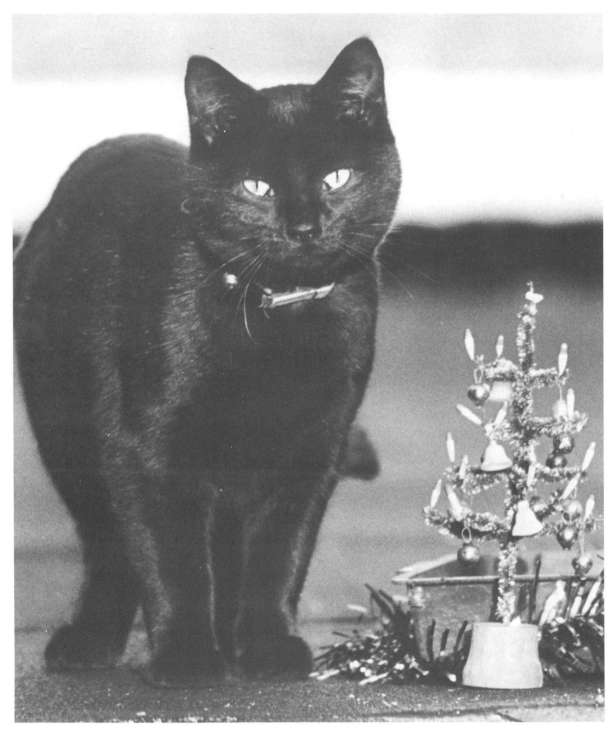

ist's widow, who left a fortune of more than £170,000 to her only companions — an elderly housekeeper, her cat Bibi, and two canaries — but nothing to her relatives, who had failed to visit her. They, of course, contested the will, which stipulated that nearly all the money was to be divided equally between the cat and the canaries, with the remainder going to the housekeeper to enable her to look after the pets in the family mansion. However, the terms of the will were upheld in court.

A complication arose when one of the two canaries slipped out of their cage, which the housekeeper had opened for cleaning, and was caught and eaten by Bibi. The relatives went to court again, this time to establish who should inherit the dead canary's share of the legacy, and whether the cat Bibi had 'lost its right of inheritance because it had murdered one of the heirs'. The court decided that a cat could not be held responsible for following its natural instincts, and that Bibi and the surviving canary should share the dead one's inheritance.

Fig 11
A working cat: Bertie, official number BM4, is one of six cats kept at the British Museum to protect priceless antiquities from the ravages of mice. His maintenance allowance is £50 per annum. Sleeping quarters and a six-foot cat-litter box are provided out of the £1.20 a year paid by each of ninety staff members.

REFERENCES

1 Langton, N. and Langton B. *The Cat in Ancient Egypt* (Cambridge University Press, 1940)
2 Manolson, Frank. *C is for Cat* (Studio Vista, 1965)

2 Food and Health

Many people may at first find it hard to believe that incorrect feeding is a common cause of illness, pain, and even deformity in cats; but unfortunately this is the case. Scientific evidence supports this statement. It is not even a matter of controversy within the veterinary profession, but proved and generally accepted, both in Britain and overseas.

The cause of such troubles is well-intentioned owners providing their cats with a virtually exclusive diet of fish, or liver, or beef, or heart.

Diet

FISH, FISH, FISH . . .

As regards an unbalanced diet, some people who themselves would never eat the same food for three meals in succession, feed their cats precisely the same food for months, sometimes years, on end, and then express surprise when the animal becomes ill.

Some cats can survive, if not thrive, on such a succession of identical meals; other cats cannot. Here are the cases of two which could not.

Case history 1. A 2½-year-old spayed cat showed symptoms of lethargy, loss of appetite, fever, and apparent pain in the back. Referred to the department of veterinary medicine, University of Bristol, it was found that the cat resented being handled, and that the inguinal (groin) fat felt lumpy. A biopsy showed that this fat was yellow. The diagnosis was **steatitis** ('yellow fat disease'). This may follow the feeding of too much oily fish such as red tuna or pilchards; but this cat's diet had, for two years, been coley. Treatment included a vitamin E supplement and a change of diet. A month later the cat was well again and no longer resisted being handled.

Case history 2. A 14-month-old neutered male, stiff in the hind legs, overweight, and with a dry, scaly coat, evinced signs of pain when its abdomen was handled. Temperature was above normal. Subcutaneous small lumps, or nodules, could be felt, as in the preceding case. The cat had been fed entirely on white fish for the previous 12 months. Again, vitamin E plus a change of diet led to a complete recovery.[1]

Note that neither of these cats had been at all well; that both had suffered pain or tenderness; and that correction of the diet enabled gradual recovery to take place. It should be emphasised, too, that steatitis does not involve merely discoloration of fat but also the death of cells and other pathological changes.

Too much fish in the diet can result also in a deficiency of thiamin (one of the B vitamins), causing a cat to become lethargic and to have a poor appetite. An unsteady gait and convulsions may occur in **Chastek paralysis** (see chapter 17) following the eating of raw fish containing a thiamin-destroying enzyme. For fish-associated **eczema**, see chapter 5.

LIVER, LIVER, LIVER . . .

The vitamin A requirement of cats is relatively greater than that of dogs research workers have pointed out; but too much vitamin A (as present in a virtually all-liver diet) may cause joint pain, lameness, and loss of appetite. After several months of regular, excessive intake of vitamin A, bony out-growths (technically known as **exostoses**) appear. In the neck so affected there is reduced potential for movement, so that the cat is to some extent crip-pled, and assumes what veterinarians call the 'angry cat' posture. The cat is in pain. The bony outgrowths may also interfere with the nerve supply to the fore-limbs. These symptoms may appear from one to five years after a cat has been on an all-liver diet, Mr David Bennett, of Glasgow University, has stated.

Liver is an excellent item of diet for the cat, to be given, say, once a fort-night, or once a week with other food, but *not every day*.

Fig 12
An alfresco meal for Chuckles, a feline friend of the author.

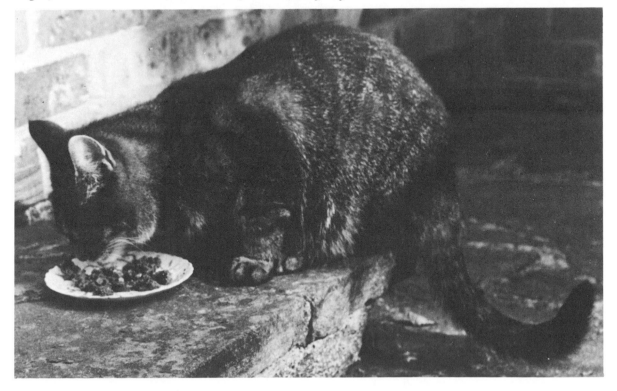

RED MEAT, RED MEAT, RED MEAT . . .

By 'red meat' in this context is meant muscle meat as opposed to offal; for example, minced beef or heart. Either of these two foods, fed continuously, can give rise to what is commonly known as the 'all-meat syndrome'. Other names are feline **juvenile osteodystrophy** or, more technically still, nutritional secondary **hypoparathyroidism**. The affected kitten becomes less playful and reluctant to jump down from even modest heights. It may become stranded when climbing curtains, owing to inability to disengage its claws. Lameness is a not uncommon symptom, and is sometimes associated with a greenstick fracture. Back pains may make a kitten bad-tempered. Deformity of the skeleton may persist in later life in such kittens as survive.

In a normal healthy animal the body maintains a correct balance between calcium and phosphorus. This calcium:phosphorus ratio is vital for health. It is upset by a virtually all red-meat diet such as minced beef or heart, because muscle contains too little calcium for the animal's needs and sufficient phosphorus to give a very adverse calcium:phosphorus ratio.

Such meat is a first-rate source of good-quality protein, and usually provides some fat too, and an excellent cat food, but *not one for every day*. (The wild cat eats virtually the whole of the carcase of its prey, so it does not suffer from this disease. Bone, skin, liver, kidney, part of the intestine and its contents, all are eaten.)

VARIETY

Most cat-owners wisely feed their animals a mixed diet, arranged to offer variety and at the same time provide the essential minerals, trace elements, and vitamins, as well as protein and carbohydrate. Variety is important not merely for the attainment of a balanced diet (and avoidance of the troubles mentioned above) but also for the sake of palatability. A monotonous diet may lead to a cat 'going off its food'.

Besides the foods already mentioned, egg, cheese, rabbit, and chicken can be incorporated into the cat's diet; likewise some boiled rice occasionally, green vegetables, and crunchy cat biscuits — if your cat will eat them.

Many, but not all cats, like milk, of course; but *fresh* drinking water should always be provided in addition.

Food should not be left down for more than half an hour, especially in warm weather. If it has not been eaten within that time, it should be removed and either put back into a refrigerator or discarded. Dishes used for cats should be kept clean; likewise drinking saucers.

CANNED FOODS

These are convenience foods, and those from reputable manufacturers are both palatable and nutritious, and carefully formulated so as to provide a

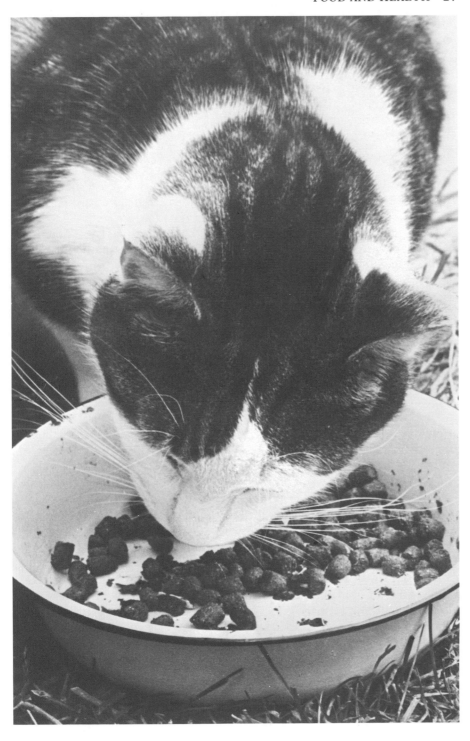

Fig 13
Food bowls and
drinking saucers
should always be kept
clean.

balanced meal. However, it is best to alternate them with some of the foods mentioned earlier rather than give them every day.

With all canned foods, the preliminary processing destroys some of the natural vitamins. Normally these are supplemented by the cat-food manufacturer, and in Britain today — as compared with the situation in the U.S.A. a few years ago, when the average levels of vitamins A, D, and E in canned cat foods were below cats' known requirements — it is very unlikely that a vitamin deficiency will occur in any of the reputable makes.

One variety of canned food can with advantage be alternated with another, so that monotony of diet is avoided. (Even if this potential for a change of flavours is ignored by a cat-owner, there is no danger — a leading manufacturer states — of a cat receiving too much liver, heart, etc., from varieties based on these ingredients, owing to the formulation.)

Cat food manufacture is big business. In 1978 the Pet Food Manufacturers' Association estimated that cats in the U.K. consumed 244,000 tonnes of canned food costing over £120 million. Cat-owners, stated the Association, spent an average of £1.01 per week on food for their animals, 80 per cent of this being prepared food, mostly canned.

Pedigree Petfoods, which has a 50 per cent share of the total U.K. pet food market, spends about £1 million per year on research and development, and employs nutritionists and veterinarians with Ph.D. degrees in this work. The company markets twelve different cat foods.

MEAT NOT FROM BUTCHERS

Previous references in this chapter to 'meat' concerned butcher's meat (i.e. that intended for human consumption) or canned cat food, and these are the only sorts which most owners ever buy for their cats. However, meat sold in slab or other form at pet stores may consist wholly or partly of knacker's meat.

There have been instances where such meat originated from a horse, cow, sheep, or goat which had been humanely 'put down' by means of a barbiturate or chloral hydrate. Cases of cats being poisoned as a result of these drugs, or of benzoic acid as a preservative, in the meat have been recorded, and though rare are worth mentioning. (See chapter 10 for instances of such poisoning.)

In the U.K. the Meat (Sterilisation) Regulations 1969 require all knacker's meat to be sterilised before being supplied to trade outlets for owners of pet animals, boarding kennels, etc. These regulations, like all regulations, may sometimes be broken or evaded, and equivalent legislation does not apply in all countries. However, the idea is to protect both the animals being fed on knacker's meat and also the housewife and her family; for even if cooked by the cat-owner before use, *unsterilised* knacker's meat can contaminate kitchen working surfaces, cook's hands, and utensils. Outbreaks of food-poisoning can arise in this way; **Salmonella** and *E. coli* organisms being most frequently involved.

Canned-meat manufacturers of repute go to great trouble to ensure efficient sterilisation of their products, and the odds must be millions to one against failure concerning any particular can or batch.

HOW MUCH, HOW OFTEN?

Cats, like people, vary in their food requirements, so that it is not possible to state precisely what any individual will need per day, to the nearest ounce. Moreover, more food will be needed in very cold weather than when it is warm; and the entire tom cat is likely to need more food than a neutered male.

As a rough guide, it is generally suggested that an average cat will need about half an ounce of food per 1 lb of bodyweight. For an adult cat, two meals per day are usually recommended, but for elderly cats it is often preferable to give smaller meals three or even four times a day. (The feeding of kittens and pregnant or nursing queens is dealt with in chapter 20.)

COOKED OR RAW?

Fish should always be cooked (and all the bones removed) before giving it to the cat. As mentioned above, thiamin is one of the vitamins necessary for cat health, and thiamin can be inactivated by an enzyme, called *thiaminase*, present in many fish. As little as 10 per cent of raw fish in the cat's diet can lead, stated Dr Lawrence Spiegel, to a thiamin deficiency.[2] Cooking destroys the harmful enzyme.

A second reason for cooking fish is the risk (mainly overseas) of fish-transmitted parasites (see chapter 6).

Should butcher's meat be fed cooked or raw? Some cat-owners favour giving it raw. Logic could be said to be on their side, for wild, as opposed to domestic, cats obviously never eat cooked meat. But they do eat their prey while the flesh is at a temperature of 90°F (33°C) or so; therefore don't forget to take your cat's meat or fish out of the refrigerator in good time. There is the additional point about flavour. People who remember to take their cheese out of the refrigerator half an hour before a meal often forget to take the cat's food out until minutes before it is going to be fed.

Maybe raw meat does have some special quality or constituent which is destroyed by cooking. On the other hand, cooked meat is safer and less likely to cause digestive upsets; and it is often said that raw meat fed to dogs and cats gives their breath an unpleasant odour.

Unless accustomed to a variable diet from kittenhood, many cats become their own worst enemies in that they decline to eat any but one, two, or possibly three different foods; but this tendency must be resisted by the owner, for reasons of feline health, and of economics, too, in some instances. Siamese, a delightful but demanding breed, have been known to opt for

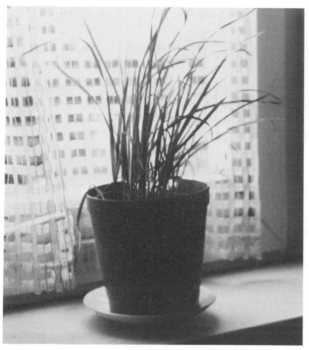

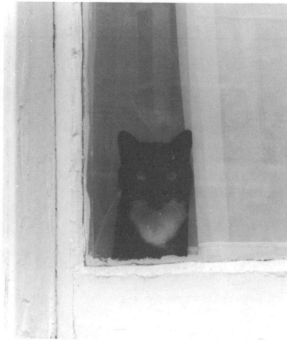

Fig 14/15
A pot of Cocksfoot grass growing on a windowsill is of benefit to a cat whose only view of the world is through a curtained window.

human food only, as opposed to cat food; and while one has never heard of any modern cat-lover buying oysters for the cat, as Dr Samuel Johnson did, they can readily become addicted to the most expensive of human luxury foods. Some cats are extremely fond of beetroot, and two greengrocers in my practice used to complain mildly that cats stole beetroot from them.

Cats normally eat a little grass, sometimes for emetic purposes; and sometimes probably as a food. Such town-dwelling cats as have no access to grass will benefit if some is grown in a pot so that they can help themselves. This is better than cutting some from a local field or park and bringing it home, because they probably will not be in the mood for it when you do. Cocksfoot seed can be obtained from the Cats Protection League, 20 North Street, Horsham, West Sussex RH12 1BN.

DANGEROUS BONES

Wild cats obtain their calcium requirements mainly from the bones of their prey, and domestic cats which do much hunting will have a similar supply. However, it is wise to remove all fish bones, chop and cutlet bones from a cat's food. Obstruction of the oesophagus or intestine by pieces of bone is far less common in the cat than in the dog, but it does occur. Similarly, pieces of bone may become wedged in the cat's mouth, causing great distress. In short, bones can be dangerous — and expensive in terms of veterinary fees, sometimes for major surgery.

A non-hunting cat which is not given bones may need a calcium supplement but, if so, this should be in the form of steamed bone flour (i.e. sterilised), and not the unsterilised bone-meal sold as a garden fertiliser.

VITAMIN SUPPLEMENTS

Essential vitamins are needed only in very small amounts, and it is easy to do harm by excessive vitamin supplementation, as explained at the beginning of this chapter. A cat receiving liver is unlikely to need a regular supplement of vitamin A. Cod-liver oil (of good quality) is an excellent source of vitamin D, and yeast is rich in the B vitamins, but with the mixed diet recommended, there is no need for the owner to worry about supplements for adult cats (other than pregnant or nursing queens) unless prescribed by a veterinary surgeon.

Health

HEREDITY AND ENVIRONMENT

Your cat's health will depend, over the years, on many different factors which

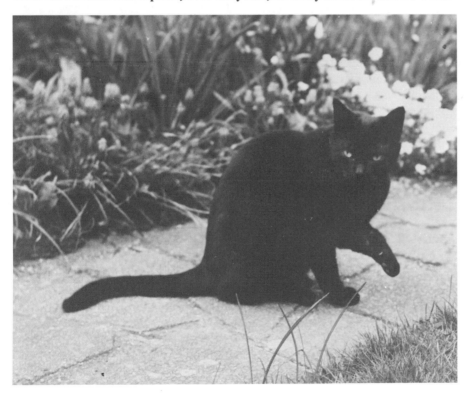

Fig 16
A good environment is an important factor for feline health, and one enjoyed by Sathi, owned by Mr and Mrs McKenzie of Ealing, and photographed when four years old.

will interact with each other, and change. First, there is what many people speak of as a 'good constitution'; and here heredity is clearly of prime importance.

Many of the most delightful cats are not 'pure-bred' and their owners have no feline pedigrees to show; yet some of these 'ordinary' cats will be more robust and healthy than some of their Show counterparts.

Breeding cats, like breeding racehorses or pedigree cattle, is an art, but even the most skilful breeders have to contend with the fact that heredity is something of a gene lottery. There may be, from the health aspect, significant differences between kittens of the same litter, even though all are sired by the same pedigree male: a situation distinct from that resulting from natural mating (i.e. not within the four walls of a pedigree cat-breeder's premises) when some kittens of the same litter may have different fathers.

After heredity comes environment. In its widest sense this means not only whether the cat has the misfortune to live in a shop in a busy town street, or the good fortune to live in a house with a large garden; but also what food the cat eats; whether it hunts in woodland or makes dangerous dashes across a road to a park; the infections it is exposed to; and the chemical substances (many harmless, some causing allergies, a few causing poisoning) with which it comes in contact. All environments have their hazards.

INFECTION AND DISEASE

Exposure of a cat to infection may or may not be followed by illness, depending on whether the cat has a useful degree of immunity against that particular infective agent; whether the animal is well nourished (and that includes its not lacking essential vitamins, minerals and trace elements in the diet); is not under stress (e.g. constantly being teased by a child, or involved in fights or overcrowding); and has not any other existing major infection, disease, or defect which might reduce its ability to resist the new infection.

Sometimes the normal immune response of the body's natural defence mechanisms may be suppressed. Some viruses can do this, e.g. the feline **leukaemia** virus.

The virulence or otherwise of the infective agent, and the quantity of it which enters the animal's body, will also have a bearing upon whether illness will follow. For example, a cat may be bitten by a rabid animal but not itself become rabid because the quantity of **rabies** virus entering the wound, from the biter's saliva, was too small and the cat's bodily defences were able to cope, which they would not have been able to do had the dose of virus been larger. (I am referring here to a cat not vaccinated against rabies.)

One must appreciate, too, that the average cat may be host to several different **parasites** at the same time. Viruses, bacteria, fungi, worms, insects, and mites — several of these may be present without the cat's owner being aware of the fact.

Cat-breeders sometimes attach scant importance to lice in kittens, over-looking the fact that a heavy infestation can cause anaemia, which may be exacerbated by worms in the intestine.

Some parasites may be too few to be causing active disease. Some, owing to the host's powers of resistance may be on the decline. Others may have a sudden opportunity for increased activity as the host's resistance becomes lowered by an additional infection, or by stress, or injury.

Case history 3. A 15-month-old short-haired cat had been abandoned, had a fight with another cat, and for a week had suffered from lack of food. A veter-inary examination showed the animal to be dehydrated as well as emaciated, with pallor of the mucous membranes. Following good feeding and admini-stration of a preparation to help reduce anaemia, the cat much improved; but two and a half weeks later became listless and lost his appetite. Laboratory tests then showed that the cat was, in fact, suffering from infectious anaemia, and his temperature fluctuated from 102.5° to 105° and then up to 106.6° on the third day of treatment, becoming normal on the sixth day. The blood parasite, *Haemobartonella felis,* responsible for the anaemia, had undoubtedly been given an opportunity to multiply owing to the stress which the cat had suffered as a result of the conditions mentioned above.[3]

A cat may encounter an infection, not become ill (or only mildly so), and develop an immunity. In other instances a cat may become ill, recover, but continue to excrete the organism. This is the 'carrier' state, in which the animal can infect other cats without showing any symptoms itself.

Some healthy cats are carriers of the feline leukaemia virus mentioned above. Some healthy Persians, for example, are carriers of ringworm.

REFERENCES

1 Flecknell, P.A. and Griffyd-Jones, T.J. *Vet. Record* 102 (1978), 149
2 Spiegel, L.S. *Petfoods Industry* (1967), 96
3 Schalm, O.W. and Switzer, J.W. *California Vet* 22 (1968), 24.

3 The Cat's Face

There is something endearing about the face of a lively, friendly cat; and its whiskers are an attractive feature. John Keats wrote:

> . . . Gaze
> With those bright languid segments green, and prick
> Those velvet ears . . .

Apart from offering a clue as to the animal's disposition, the face of a cat also provides some indication of its state of health. The veterinary surgeon notes at a glance whether the eyes are bright and lustrous, as they should be; whether the third eyelid is prominent; whether the nose is free from discharge, the lips free of saliva, the fur clean-looking and glossy. Is there a bald patch anywhere? Several skin diseases appear first on the head.

The Eyelids

Each of the eyelids is lined by a mucous membrane, the conjunctiva. This forms small pockets and it is in these that grass awns or particles of grit sometimes lodge, leading to inflammation. This **conjunctivitis** leads, as we all

Fig 17
Eye examination. A veterinary surgeon using an ophthalmoscope.

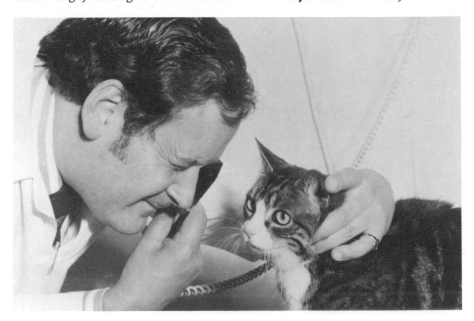

know from personal experience, to 'watering' of the eyes, often to inflammation also of the edges of the eyelids; sometimes to a sticky, thicker discharge. There may be tenderness or pain, and a reluctance to keep the eyes open in a bright light.

Conjunctivitis may arise from a purely local infection, or it may be one symptom of a generalised illness such as '**Cat flu**'.

Numerous micro-organisms can infect a cat's eye, including *Chlamydia* and *Moraxella*.

Case history. An outbreak of Moraxella infection occurred in a cattery, and affected 90 per cent of the inmates: 23 adult cats and 30 kittens. The outbreak lasted nine weeks. Although the conjunctivitis was severe, the cats did not lose their liveliness.[1]

Cats, like people, can suffer from an allergy, with conjunctivitis and sneezing, as seen in 'hay fever'.

'Watering' of one eye may be the result of blockage of a tear duct, or of a foreign body in the conjunctival pocket. If a tear duct is blocked, reddish-brown tear staining of any white fur may occur. The discoloration is due to a pigment in the lacrimal fluid (tears).

Turning in of the eyelids (**entropion**) is rare in the cat.

THE THIRD EYELIDS

The nictitating membrane, or third eyelid, situated at the inner angle of the eye, normally has little more than its edge exposed to view. Its appearance,

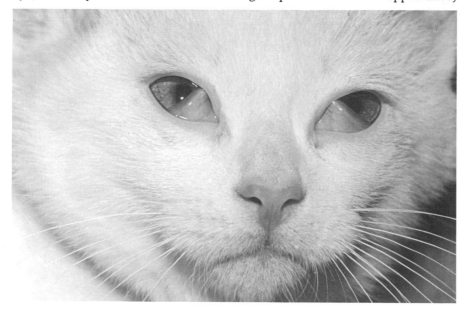

Fig 18
The *membrana nictitans* ('third eyelid') partly covering each eye. Usually this follows absorption of orbital fat during illness, but this cat was apparently in good health.

like curtains partly drawn across a window, is often an important indicator of the cat's general health. True, it may be an accompaniment of conjunctivitis or other local eye disorder; but in the absence of these it is usually a sign of debility. For example, the cat may be anaemic, or have some viral infection, or be losing weight.

The Eyes

Inflammation of the cornea — the eye's window, so to speak, which admits light through the pupil to the retina — is known as **keratitis**. This may be the result of infection, or penetration by another cat's claw or by a thorn.

Symptoms include the profuse watering of the eye and a tendency to keep the eyes closed as seen with severe conjunctivitis, but then there follows an opacity which at first may be only pin-head size. This is sometimes the clue to the presence of a thorn embedded in the eye. The thorn itself rarely attracts the owner's attention, but the tiny circle of white around the thorn is readily noticed. A thorn must be removed under anaesthesia by a veterinary surgeon.

Keratitis rarely involves the whole of a cat's cornea; but should it do so, the animal will be temporarily blind. **Pannus** is a complication of keratitis in which blood-vessels run in from its margin, e.g. towards any ulcer which may be present. Occasionally an ulcer penetrates the cornea, and there may be a hernia of part of the iris. The cornea may be penetrated too by a shotgun pellet. **Scleritis** is inflammation of the sclera or 'white of the eye' and gives the bloodshot appearance.

A **cataract**, or cloudy appearance of the lens, may form in a diabetic or elderly cat, impairing vision. Some veterinary surgeons specialising in ophthalmic surgery do remove lenses, whether dislocated or opaque from cataract, but the operation is seldom called for in respect of the cat.

There are many other abnormal eye conditions, some due to hereditary factors, e.g. a squint; some due to diet, e.g. a deficiency of vitamin A; some due to infections which involve the retina or optic nerve, e.g. **toxoplasmosis**, feline leukaemia.

Euthanasia is the only humane solution to the problem of a cat which has become totally blind; but enucleation of one damaged eye is well justified since cats make good recoveries from this operation in nearly all cases and apparently enjoy life afterwards. No ugly, gaping socket is left after the operation, which leaves no trace of where the eye has been.

The Nose

In health the nostrils should be free from discharge and, equally, not dry and cracked. Catarrhal inflammation of the nose, and also sinusitis, are described in chapter 12, 'The Sneezing Cat' (see also chapter 8, 'Nursing').

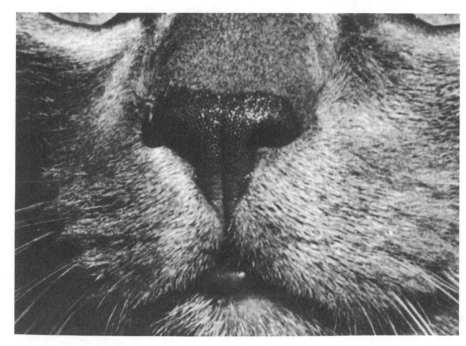

Fig 19
The nose of a cat.

Facial Swellings

One of the commonest causes is an abscess, often following a bite from another cat. A sinus or 'hole' which fails to heal may be due to an infected tooth; the pus having taken this escape route to the skin surface. Extraction of such a tooth will allow permanent healing to take place. Swelling of the parotid glands may be due to **mumps**. In other instances a tumour may alter the shape of the face.

The Ears

One of these may assume a crinkled appearance after being ballooned out by a **haematoma** on the inside of the pinna or flap (see chapter 11). **Ear mange** is described in chapter 5; also the complications which may follow neglected cases. Occasionally a **tumour** grows within the ear; for example a benign tumour which has a stalk and is called a **polyp**. This can be removed surgically and is unlikely to recur. A malignant growth known as a **ceruminous adenocarcinoma**, rarely found in any animal but the cat, is so seldom seen that mention of it here should not alarm the cat-owner.

The ear flaps are often the first places to be affected by **notoedric mange**, when bald patches may appear.

Deafness can be a congenital defect, and is one for a buyer to be wary of if choosing a white cat, especially if it has blue eyes. Temporary deafness may be due to carbon monoxide poisoning. Permanent deafness may follow injury to an ear-drum, blockage of the Eustachian tube, a nerve or brain injury, or pressure from a tumour on these. Loss of hearing often occurs in elderly cats.

The Chin

This is not uncommonly the site of an acne-like condition. The fur becomes matted with discharge from the pustules. This condition does not yield readily to first-aid measures, and professional treatment should be obtained.

The Mouth

Disorders affecting the mouth are dealt with in chapter 15, 'Digestive System Disorders', but it seems appropriate to refer here to the inability of a cat to close its mouth, since this will alter the normal appearance of the face. Among likely causes is displacement of a loose tooth in an older cat, a foreign body wedged in the mouth or, far less commonly, dislocation or fracture of the jaws. The lower jaw may hang open in cases of rabies also. The cat's appearance may be altered, too, by an **epulis** or tumour affecting the gum. The lip is sometimes the site of an ulcer which tends to spread despite first-aid measures, and also becomes deep. Professional treatment should be obtained.

Fig 20
Healthy teeth and gums.

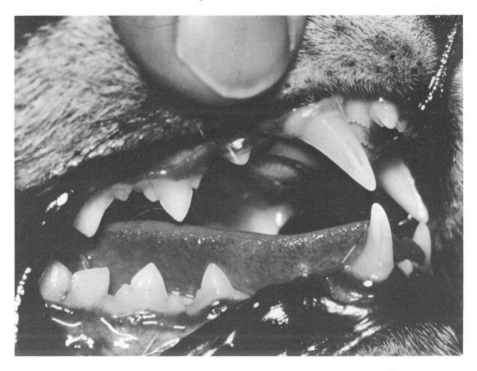

The Teeth

The number of teeth in the adult cat averages 30. They comprise, in the upper jaw, 6 incisors, 2 canine teeth, 6 premolars, and 2 molars; while the lower jaw has 6 incisors, 2 canines, 4 premolars, and 2 molars. Some cats have only 28 permanent teeth, lacking 2 premolars.

When the teeth of middle-aged or elderly cats have been neglected, tartar may attain considerable bulk, forming hard masses over several teeth which are completely covered and masked. Their appearance suggests almost that the teeth have become joined together and assumed a different shape. This and other tooth disorders are discussed in chapter 15.

REFERENCES

1 Withers, A.R. and Davies, M.E. *Vet. Record* 73 (1961), 858

4 Skin, Fur, Claws and Paws

Skin and Fur

The skin is, of course, a protective covering for the body, and consists of two main layers. The outer of these (the *epidermis*) has a hard, dry surface part, with flat plate-like cells which flake off to form scurf; and a deeper, soft, moist part with cells multiplying and being gradually pushed upwards, away from the blood vessels in the deeper, second part (the *corium*, or *dermis*) until they too flatten, die, and flake off.

The corium consists of a network of fibrous tissue, including elastic fibres, well supplied with blood vessels, and containing the hair follicles, sebaceous glands, lymph vessels, and nerves. The topmost layer of the corium is dovetailed, so to speak, into the epidermis by ridges and nipple-like projections.

Each hair of the cat's fur has a shaft — the visible part — and a root embedded in the hair follicle. The whiskers have follicles which are abundantly supplied with nerves. Hairs are pigmented, giving to the coat its characteristic colour. Special muscles enable hairs to be erected when the cat is angry, afraid, or very cold.

As well as protecting the body, skin and hair assist in the heat regulation processes which normally maintain a constant body temperature. Cats can be regarded as non-sweating animals. It is true that sweat glands can be found in the skin; but only from the pads of the feet is cooling achieved in this way for all practical purposes. Panting is not a normal method of body cooling in the cat, as it is in the dog, and is a danger signal. Excess heat may induce a flow of watery saliva which the cat spreads on its fur; evaporation then effects cooling.

The cat's fur, and especially the air trapped in it, provides insulation against cold. In very low temperatures the hairs can be erected. Shivering may also occur. If it does, heat will be produced. However, in extremes of cold, or under anaesthesia, shivering may cease, and **hypothermia** ensue.

A heat-regulation centre in the brain is able to influence the rate of metabolism, constrict or dilate surface blood vessels and bring about the effects mentioned; but in extremes of temperature it may be unable to cope. Heat exhaustion and heat stroke are referred to in chapter 9, since **hyperthermia** constitutes an emergency. It may occur under adverse travelling conditions, and the cat's body temperature may rise from its normal 101-101.5° to 107° or more. The cat *will* be panting, in all probability, and unless the temperature is quickly brought down, the animal will lapse into a coma, probably have convulsions, and die. First-aid consists in applications of cold water to the cat's body.

Hyperthermia can affect unborn kittens, as explained in chapter 20, without causing obvious symptoms in the queen.

The opposite state, hypothermia, may occur in a cat suffering from exposure, accidentally trapped in a cold store, etc., as well as during anaesthesia.

SKIN DISORDERS

Being on the outside, the skin is naturally exposed to damage by violence, parasites, chemical irritants, extremes of temperature, and to what Professor I.A. Silver M.A., M.R.C.V.S., University of Bristol Medical School, has described as 'misdirection of normal protective responses, e.g. allergic reactions'.

Like muscles, the skin can atrophy, or over-develop (**hypertrophy**), and can show abnormalities in its formation. Like all tissues, the skin may be the site of benign or malignant tumours.

As we all appreciate, a glossy coat in a smooth-coated cat is one of the signs of good health, whereas a lustreless appearance suggests that all is not well and may indicate an insufficiency of fat in the diet, a vitamin deficiency, the presence of worms in the intestine or of external parasites, or disease of the kidneys.

Parting the fur one can see whether the skin is clean, scurfy, dry, or oily, and whether it is of normal colour and appearance. In cases of **seborrhoea** there may be an abnormal amount of scurf, and sometimes a greasy skin. An abnormal odour is present in some skin diseases and some illnesses.

MOULTING

The hairs are constantly being shed and replaced by others, though the extent to which this occurs and becomes noticeable may be greater in the spring and autumn, when more frequent grooming is advisable. There is no cause for alarm at the quantity shed provided that the skin remains covered; i.e. there are no bald patches.

FELTING

Regular grooming is essential for long-haired breeds such as Persians and for those with coats of medium length. Unfortunately it is not carried out by some owners, with the result that large lumps of a felt-like consistency are formed. These have to be *cut* away — a painstaking task — as combing is by

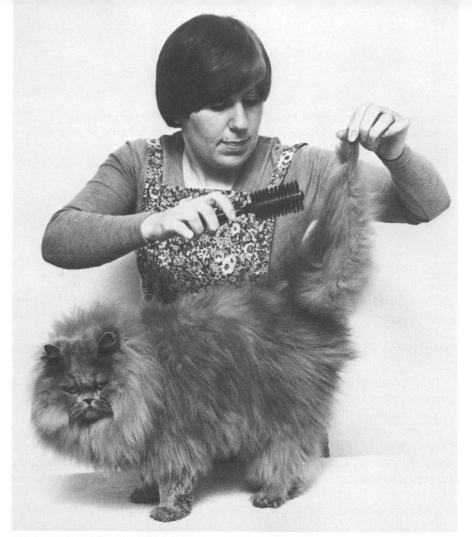

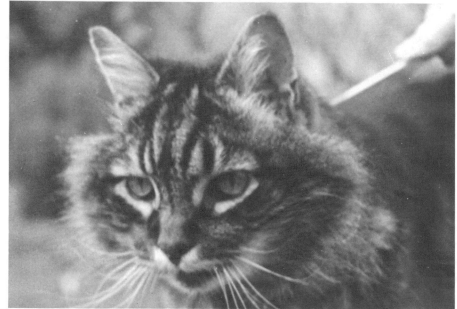

Fig 21
The regular grooming
of long-haired cats is
essential, and they
should be accustomed
to it from an early age.
Fig 22
Kim, having jumped
on to the stool to be
combed, is now
enjoying it. He was
over 17 when photo-
graphed by the author,
and is a credit to Mrs
E.M. Deacon and Miss
R.M.A. Turner.

then impossible and for fractious cats an anaesthetic may be required.

Grooming is an essential part of parasite control, and cats should be accustomed to it from an early age. This is often easier said than done, because many Persians, for instance, resist fiercely, and they are the ones most in need of grooming. Many cats, on the other hand, welcome grooming and will jump on to a stool in pleasurable anticipation and purr when grooming begins.

COAT COLOUR

People will tell you that all ginger cats are male, and all tortoiseshell cats are female. While this is certainly true of the vast majority, nevertheless the 'rule' is not absolute. (see chapter 19).

It is well known that Siamese kittens are born white, and later develop the cream body-colour with the chocolate-hued face, ears, feet and tail — the so-called points. Probably less well known, however, is the fact that these changes are influenced by temperature. White hairs may appear among the dark ones after a fever. Siamese which spend much time outdoors in the colder parts of the U.S.A., for example, tend to be darker. The fur grows back darker after a cat's abdomen has been shaved preparatory to surgery, and similarly at the site of an abscess.

The influence of temperature on Siamese coat colour changes was studied by two Moscow scientists, N.A. and U.N. Iljix, and published in a 1930 issue of the *Journal of Heredity*. Dr Donald Innes,[1] a Californian veterinarian who drew attention to their work (which provided experimental proof), also demonstrated the effect of a bandage on a Siamese cat.

In America methylene blue was at one time used, in conjunction with other compounds, as a urinary antiseptic. However, it is unsafe for cats, not only

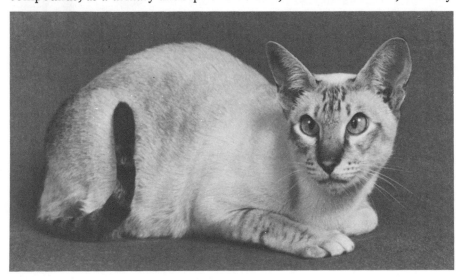

Fig 23
Siamese – Seal Tabby Point.

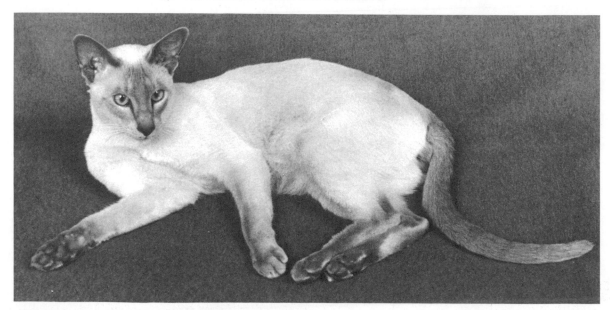

Fig 24
A Lilac-Point Siamese.
Fig 25
In some circumstances,
a bath does become
necessary.

causing the skin and fur of a white cat to take on a bluish tinge, but also giving rise to **Heinz-body anaemia**, which can prove fatal.

Badly soiled and matted fur around the anus — a very unhygienic and malodorous condition likely to occur in long-haired cats suffering from diarrhoea — needs attention. If neglected, the cat will in many cases be unable to empty its rectum, and become very distressed; also, during summer, matters may be complicated by blowflies and their maggots. The use of scissors (never use sharp-pointed ones but always ones with curved ends) and a tepid, diluted antiseptic solution for use on cotton wool are indicated. TCP, Milton, hydrogen peroxide, or a teaspoonful of common salt in a pint of water are all safe for use on cats.

BATHING

Cats being fastidious creatures which wash themselves nearly all over (they cannot reach the back of their necks or between their shoulder blades), the question of bathing them does not arise except: (1) in cases of a severe infestation with external parasites which have been allowed to become very numerous; for example, neglected mange, a coat which is full of fleas and flea excrement, or lice; (2) as a first-aid measure when a cat has fallen into some poisonous liquid or become smeared with it; (3) as a first-aid treatment for heat stroke or heat stress; (4) for a very few old cats which have ceased to wash themselves; (5) for entire tom cats which have been closely confined and, as a result of stress or illness, have become in need of a bath since they, too, have ceased to look after themselves.

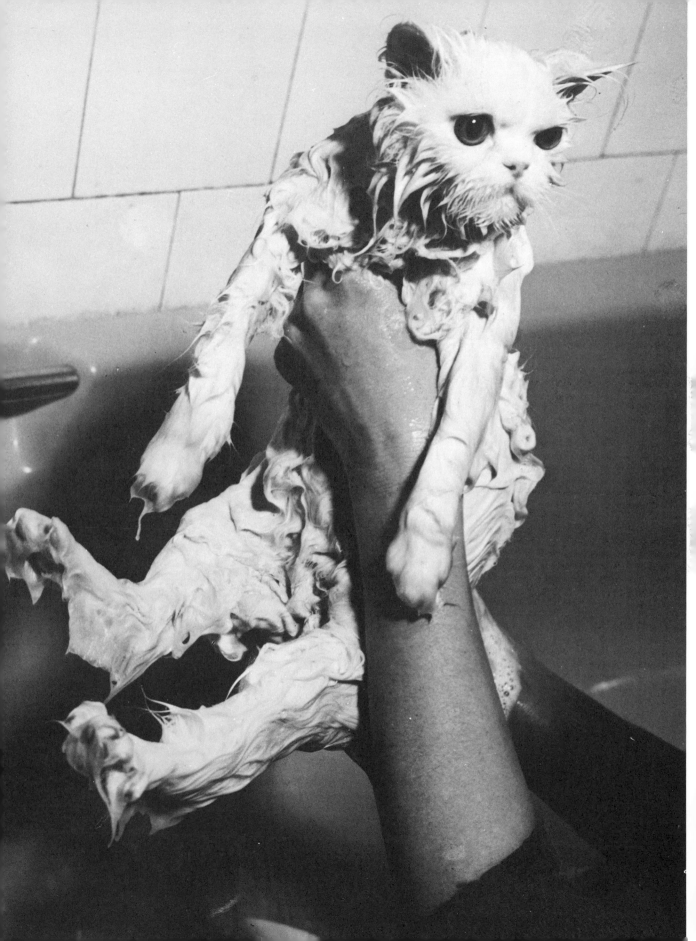

ALOPECIA

Some veterinarians refer to all bald patches as **alopecia**; but most use the term in a restricted sense, excluding loss of fur due to external parasites, eczema, scalds and burns, and reserving it mainly for the results of nutritional deficiencies, hormone imbalances, and the effects of poisons such as selenium and thallium.

Congenital alopecia is not unknown in cats, and there may well be a hereditary predisposition to some alopecias.

Fig 26
A bare, scaly patch on a kitten's toe due to ringworm – transmissible to man.

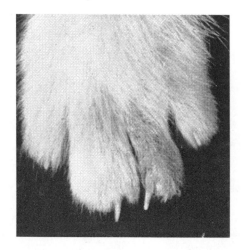

Mange, ringworm, and eczema (described in chapter 5) all have to be differentiated by the veterinary surgeon, when forming his diagnosis, from bare patches due to other causes.

A hormone imbalance (excess of one particular hormone in relation to another) often produces bald patches which are symmetrical, i.e. they occur on both sides of the body. It is often possible to correct such imbalances, and restore fur growth. A deficiency of thyroid gland hormone, or of the trace element iodine, causes alopecia in cats of both sexes. In spayed and castrated cats, problems sometimes arise.

Senile alopecia is a recognised condition in the cat.

The Paws

The normal cat has five toes on the fore feet, and four on the hind feet. (The term *polydactyl* is applied to cats which have extra toes; e.g. six on the fore feet and five on the hind feet.)

The skin between the toes may become inflamed as a result of the cat stepping in some irritating substance, e.g. petrol, motor oil, tar, and perhaps making matters worse by frantic licking. Sometimes a grass seed or awn, or a small piece of road grit, becomes lodged there, and may penetrate the skin, causing an abscess.

Harvest mites, visible as bright orange/red specks, may cause intense irritation in the space between the toes.

Thorns or pieces of broken glass may similarly cause damage to the skin of the interdigital space, or may penetrate the pads. With a deep cut, sutures may have to be applied by a veterinary surgeon to draw the edges of the wound together; otherwise healing may be very protracted. Occasionally bleeding from such a cut is alarming.

As a first-aid measure, before taking the cat to a veterinary surgery, an attempt may be made to apply a bandage. First take a large piece of cotton wool, and wrap it round the leg to include the paw. Then apply the bandage, not too tightly, over the cotton wool. (Tight bandaging of the leg or foot, with no cotton wool to provide a cushioning effect can be dangerous, and should never be carried out, since it interferes too much with the circulation.)

The cat may remove the bandage in much less time than you and your helper took to put it on; but at least you will have tried.

The Claws

A cat's claws are derived from the same layer of cells in the developing embryo as the skin and fur; and as with the skin, the hard outer part of the claw is composed of modified epidermis, and the soft, sensitive, inner part — the quick — of corium.

Just as a hair grows from its follicle, so the claw grows from its matrix, which is supplied by blood vessels and nerves. Extending into the matrix is a projection of the third phalanx bone.

Occasionally dew-claws need attention if they are growing in a circle and penetration of the skin is threatened; loose and hanging dew-claws may be surgically removed under anaesthesia by a veterinary surgeon should they be troubling the cat.

Normally, nail trimming is required only in unweaned kittens to protect their mother, or in an adult cat that has been closely confined for some time (perhaps to aid healing of a fracture), or in very old age: cats benefit in each instance.

From the owner's point of view, taking the sharp points off a cat's claws before dressing a wound, bathing, or giving other attention likely to be resented, is a sensible precaution and avoids bloodshed — unless the cat is of a very aggressive disposition and will not permit claw-tips to be trimmed.

Claw-trimming must be done with care. With unpigmented claws, the quick is visible as a pink core, and this is a guide as to how far it is safe to cut. Always allow a short space of solid claw between the sensitive quick and where you cut, or you will hurt the cat.

With pigmented claws, the quick may be hard to see or completely invisible, one must therefore proceed cautiously, cutting too little rather than too much.

INJURED CLAWS

Sometimes a claw becomes torn or broken. If only the solid part is involved, there is no need to interfere, and new growth of horn will repair the damage. If the claw is broken higher up, exposing the sensitive quick, the part will be painful. The claw is likely to slough off, a new claw eventually replacing the lost one.

Fig 27
The roughened appearance of an infected claw. *Microsporum canis* Bodin was responsible in each case.

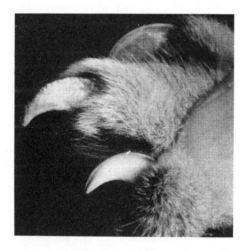

Infection sometimes follows an injury, with pus visible or oozing at the junction of claw and skin when pressed very gently. With most cats, it is best to seek professional help; but should yours be amenable to first-aid, you can try putting the whole paw into a big jam jar containing warm saline (a teaspoonful of kitchen salt to a pint of water). It needs one person to hold the jar firmly, while the other copes with the cat and holds the paw in the water. Pain and swelling can both be relieved by this means, *if* the cat does not struggle or resort to use of tooth and (undamaged) claw.

Some cases of claw infection are due to one or other of the fungi causing ringworm.

DE-CLAWING

The exercising of the cat's claw muscles — usually referred to as claw sharpening — cannot always be prevented by providing an old mat or even a piece of tree trunk. Sometimes a Siamese, for instance, will choose for the purpose some highly expensive wallpaper. This has led to the demand by owners for a de-clawing operation. 'This is considered in the same light as neutering in North America,' commented Mr Peter Randell in the *Veterinary Record*.

> Our cat was de-clawed when six months old, at the same time as castration, and now he is six. The saving in undamaged furniture is incalculable. In climbing he obtains all his purchase with his hind feet; in fighting he will acquit himself well with any tom. (It seems that by nature cats are somewhat over-armed.) He still goes through the motions of sharpening his front claws without any apparent loss of emotional satisfaction.

The British Veterinary Association's policy on de-clawing was made clear in a statement issued in June 1979. 'The removal of claws in felines is undesirable and should be carried out in extreme circumstances only, when the alternative is euthanasia.'

REFERENCES

1 Innes, Donald C. *Feline Practice* 3 (1977), 27.

5 The Itchy Cat

Parasites

FLEAS

If a cat is scratching or nibbling its fur, the most likely cause is the presence of fleas, since these are the most common external parasites. Capable of fast movement, they are dark brown in colour and have very narrow bodies (i.e. they are tall and thin). These insects have mouth parts adapted for piercing the skin and sucking blood.

Some cat-owners seem to find it shaming to be told that their cat has fleas, though why this is so is a little puzzling. Any but the most closely confined cat is bound to acquire fleas sooner or later; it is only when they are knowingly allowed to remain that the cat-owner need feel self-critical. Other owners readily accept the fact that their cats have fleas, but are unaware of the threat caused to the cat's health.

At the beginning of an infestation a few fleas may not greatly trouble the cat or result in scratching frequent enough to attract the owner's attention. As the number of fleas increases, however, the itchiness interferes with the cat's rest, and blood loss may begin to become significant. Moreover, some cats become sensitised to the flea's saliva, which enters into the bite wounds. When this has occurred, only one or two fleas are sufficient in the hypersensitive cat to provoke a distressing allergic reaction: one type of eczema. **Pruritus** (itchiness) is intense, and the cat may bite and scratch itself until blood is drawn by its claws and bald patches may appear among the fur. Secondary infection may occur, with further discomfort.

The cat has its own species of flea — one which, it seems, thrives in homes with central heating, whereas the latter provides conditions less favourable to the life-cycle of the human flea, which is better suited by a cold, damp environment. Flea infestations can be mixed ones. (In a survey of flea-infested dogs in Dublin it was found that 128 had dog fleas only; 24 dogs were infested entirely by the human flea; 12 by both dog and human fleas; 4 by cat fleas; and 2 by both dog and cat fleas.)

All these species of flea may bite people — another reason for not tolerating continuing flea infestation of your cat. Then again, fleas transmit tapeworm larvae, the cat becoming host to an adult tapeworm after swallowing an infected flea.

A cat heavily infested with fleas will have a dirty skin. If the fur is parted, blackish dots of flea excrement may be seen, and fleas will not be hard to find.

Fleas do not breed on their host, as lice do. Flea eggs are laid on the cat's bedding, or on the floor of a room. Larvae emerge from the hatched eggs, develop in stages, and later the adult flea emerges from a pupa.

Ridding a cat of its fleas involves two separate courses of action: (1) killing the fleas on the cat's body by means of a dry shampoo, aerosol spray, 'flea-collar', or wet shampoo; and (2) destruction of existing bedding material (if used), and attention to places where flea eggs may hatch (e.g. cracks between floorboards, carpeting, skirting boards, cracks in woodwork or, in catteries, concrete). Dry cat shampoo powder may be put down in such places. In catteries a flame-gun may be used. In the modern living-room thorough vacuum cleaning will gather up most of the flea eggs and larvae. Re-infestation will inevitably occur if this second course of action is neglected.

Insecticidal shampoo powders can be bought at pet shops, but choose one of a reputable make, and be sure that 'suitable for use on cats' is included in the wording on the packet. The same advice applies to the purchase of aerosol spray cans. Always use these preparations strictly in accordance with the manufacturer's instructions.

DDT preparations must never be used on cats (see chapter 10); and B.H.C. preparations, excellent for canine use, are risky for cats and best avoided.

De-fleaing may conveniently be carried out on a table covered with news-paper. Apply a little of the aerosol spray or the dry shampoo powder to the root of the tail, and then some at the back of the cat's head and neck (taking care that none gets on to the face). Powder must be rubbed gently in among the fur. Then apply more of the insecticide along the back and flanks.

Hold the cat for as long as practicable, to prevent licking; then comb out the powder and dead or dying fleas on to the newspaper, and burn it.

'Flea-collars' of a reputable make are effective against fleas, lice, and ticks over a period of, say, 7 – 12 weeks. Many owners are fearful of any collar on account of the risk of a cat being caught by a branch or other projection while out hunting. However, a flea-collar could be put on at night and taken off in the morning. When flea-collars are worn for long periods, a watch should be kept for any signs of inflammation of the skin, as a few cats may become allergic to the insecticide.

In a survey carried out in America by *Feline Practice*, most of the 20 responding veterinarians considered that 'the benefits far outweighed the risks'. Neck dermatitis occurred, it was stated, in between 1 and 5 per cent of cats wearing these collars — often because they were applied too tightly. It was advised that the collar, when adjusted, should be loose enough to admit two fingers between it and the cat's neck. It helped, some veterinarians pointed out, if the cat were accustomed to an ordinary cat collar before application of a flea collar. *Warnings:* do not use these on young kittens; if a cat comes in wet, remove the flea-collar and do not re-apply until dry. In *bad* cases, redness and loss of fur might extend in a circle around the neck.

Wet shampoos are available, but again not all are safe for cats, so heed the advice offered above. The cat will probably resent being given a bath, but if the water is warm, not hot, will usually suffer the indignity without inflicting scratches on its owner.

Wet shampoos are probably best reserved for very bad infestations with parasites such as fleas and lice, or for *Cheyletiella* mites which, owing to their tunnelling among skin débris, are resistant to insecticide applied in powder or aerosol form.

Selenium sulphide washes, sold under various proprietary names, are suitable and safer than B.H.C. Rinsing is necessary afterwards.

Finally, before leaving the subject of fleas, one should mention the 'stick-tight' or chicken flea, which may infest a cat after it has caught a wild bird. The female flea attaches its mouth parts to the skin, often of the cat's ear, and remains there, tightly secured.

LICE

Without a good light and a magnifying glass, lice are hard to see. Whereas a flea, with its dark brown colour, attracts the eye, the greyish louse merges into its background. The eggs or 'nits' are laid on the host, are white, and each is attached to a hair. The louse's whole life-cycle takes place on its host.

Lice can multiply rapidly, and a severe infestation may cause not only great irritation but an anaemia which can be serious in a debilitated adult cat and may prove fatal in a kitten (especially one infested also with worms). Lice can also transmit tapeworm larvae and other parasites.

While lice are readily killed by shampoos effective against fleas, their eggs or 'nits' are not; accordingly it is essential to repeat the treatment in a fortnight's time, or to give three treatments at 10-day intervals. Severe infestation of long-haired cats may require some clipping of the fur if this has become at all matted.

TICKS

These parasites may be found on town cats as well as those living in the country. All the ticks likely to be encountered in Britain are three-host ticks; that is to say, the larva, nymph, and adult each feeds on a different animal, dropping off after doing so. They climb up blades of grass, etc, and attach themselves to a passing animal.

A single tick may be found on a cat's head, for example, or two or three; sometimes several small larval ticks around the lips. To anyone unfamiliar with ticks, an engorged female may look more like a small tumour than a parasite, since mouth-parts and legs will be hidden under its body, as the illustration shows. Once recognised, a tick must be removed. This may be facilitated by applying a drop of surgical spirit or lighter-fuel to the tick, and

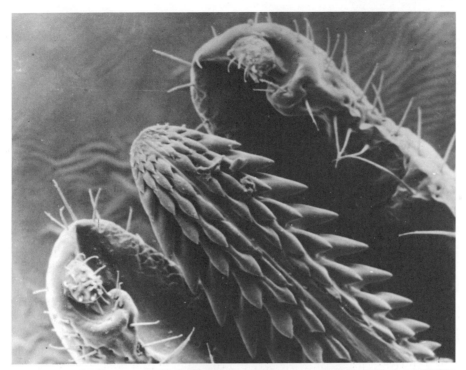

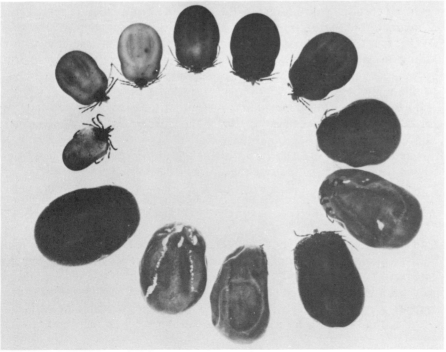

Fig 28
The mouth parts of a tick.
Fig 29
Various stages (clockwise from centre left) in the engorgement of a female tick. When engorged, mouth parts and legs are concealed, so that the tick may not be recognised as a parasite at all.

waiting a little. The parasite may withdraw its mouth-parts from the cat's skin and back away. It can then be removed with forceps or tweezers. If it is merely pulled, the mouth-parts may break off and be left embedded in the skin, sometimes resulting in an abscess.

Ticks cause local inflammation, some secrete a toxin; all suck blood and worry the host.

While ticks can be removed by hand, or killed by means of a wet shampoo, there is no effective tick-deterrent which can be used. A 'flea-collar' — while not deterring ticks from climbing on to a cat — will kill them once they are there.

EAR MANGE

This is the most common cause of a cat shaking its head or scratching its ears, and is caused by *Otodectes* mites (which also infest dogs' ears). The names **ear mange** or **parasitic otitis** are preferable to the word 'canker' which is used by owners indiscriminately to describe a variety of different ear troubles.

Inside the outer ear a deposit of waxy-powdery material will be present, brown or blackish in colour. When this is examined under a microscope or a powerful magnifying glass, the mites can be seen.

As a first-aid measure, a little medicinal liquid paraffin or cooking oil may be allowed to trickle into the ear, and this may help to soften the deposit.

On no account poke around in the ear with cotton wool 'fastened' to an orange stick or tweezers, or serious and painful damage may be caused. Avoid, too, filling the ears with 'canker powder', which may clog without killing the mites. Instead, obtain from your veterinary surgeon ear drops appropriate for the actual condition present in *your* cat. A safe mite-killer will be one ingredient.

If a bacterial or fungal infection is present, or the ear is ulcerated and painful, different ear drops can be supplied to relieve the pain and overcome infection.

It is unkind to the cat to leave ear mange untreated. The constant head shaking and scratching indicate the animal's discomfort.

NOTOEDRIC MANGE

Caused by the parasitic mite *Notoedres cati,* notoedric mange is the feline equivalent of sarcoptic mange in the dog and is intensely irritating. A typical case begins on the ears and quickly spreads to the face. Neck, elbows and feet may soon be affected, too. As the fur falls out, the skin in the bald areas appears greyish and scurfy. In neglected cases there is wrinkling and thickening of the skin. Self-inflicted wounds cause further damage and facilitate secondary infection.

Diagnosis is confirmed, when necessary, by taking skin scrapings and, after suitable preparation, examining them under the microscope, when the mites can be recognised.

With cats, as already mentioned, there is a very limited choice of parasiticides which can be used without risk of poisoning. Fortunately, however, in most parts of Britain — if not all — notoedric mange seems to have become a rarity.

HARVEST MITES

The so-called 'harvest mite' or 'chigger' is the larva of *Trombicula autumnalis*, and the cause of intense itching in man, cat, dog, and other creatures. Before burrowing under the skin, it may be seen as a speck of orange or orange-red. The infestation remains a local one; sometimes between the toes.

CHEYLETIELLA MITES

These infest people, rabbits, hares, foxes, dogs, and cats. The latter probably suffer less than the other animals owing to their habit of washing themselves. Itching varies from mild to intense; the parasites congregating usually along the back, sometimes on the head and neck. As mentioned earlier, a selenium preparation is suitable for treatment, but must be rinsed out afterwards.

Eczema

This is an inflammatory condition of the skin and takes various forms; e.g. 'wet eczema', which has a bright red, moist appearance; and 'dry eczema', which has a scaly, dry appearance. Itchiness often accompanies eczema and at times may provoke almost frantic licking.

Some cases are the result of an allergy, and the cat becoming hypersensitised to flea's saliva has already been mentioned. It is one of the commonest causes or contributory factors, and so a search for fleas must be made. Other individual allergies are said to result from substances present in carpets, rubber, fabrics. Eczema has often been linked with an almost exclusively fish diet, which should be changed. A lack of vitamin A may be a contributory factor. Diseases of the kidneys may be associated with some cases of eczema; possibly diabetes. In some spayed females and castrated males a hormone imbalance is another factor which, together with faulty diet and fleas, or on its own account, is of importance. Hormone treatment — including the implant of a long-lasting pellet of testosterone in the castrated male — is often successful.

Veterinary treatment with an anti-histamine will often relieve the itching due to an allergy. Calamine lotion is soothing, but has to be used with care or it will be licked off.

Ringworm

This is a fungal disease mainly of young cats; older ones have greater resistance. The fungus *Microsporum canis* is responsible for most cases of cat ringworm, *Trichophyton* species for a few cases, and others may be involved too.

The first-named species does not cause much itchiness as a rule, but the second does. It is the appearance of a small bare patch which usually attracts the owner's attention. If closely examined, the hairs will be seen to have been broken off, and the skin shows greyish scales. The patches, often raised at their edges, are most commonly seen on the head and legs. Ringworm is at times a misnomer because the lesions are not always circular: they may be irregular in shape to begin with, or they may be circular at first but, as the disease spreads, and affected areas coalesce, the outline may become anything but circular. **Mycotic dermatitis** or **dermatomycosis** are accordingly names often preferred in textbooks to ringworm.

The cat's claws are a common ringworm site, and instead of a smooth surface there may be a roughness visible. This claw infection is known as **Onychomosis**.

Favus is a name for what is sometimes colloquially known as 'honey-comb' ringworm, characterised by cup-shaped crusts. Cats may become infected with favus by rats and mice.

Diagnosis of ringworm depends for its confirmation on laboratory methods: microscopic examination of skin scrapings, suitably treated; or the use of a Wood's lamp. Under the latter — a source of ultra-violet light — many *but not all* of the fungi (depending on species and strain) will fluoresce in a

Fig 30
A cat with ringworm, caused by the fungus *Microsporum canis*. This is not, however, a typical case of the disease.
Fig 31 (right) Another case of ringworm, more typical in appearance than the first. The greyish-whitish, scaly lesion can be seen to the right of the ear, above the white fur.

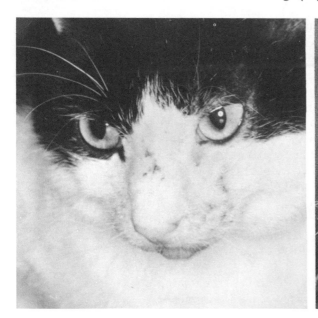

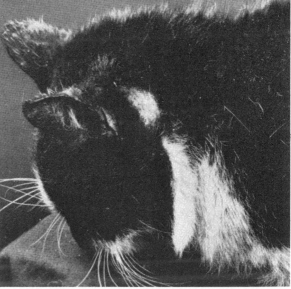

dark room.

Treatment is by one of two means: (1) giving an antibiotic, griseofulvin, in the cat's food. This is an expensive antibiotic, but very convenient, especially where several cats are involved, as in boarding catteries, for example. The method obviates much otherwise necessary handling of infected cats, and so reduces the risk of human infection occurring. However, in breeding catteries, griseofulvin must not be given to pregnant queens, or deformed kittens may result. (2) A local application to the site of the ringworm of a safe and suitable fungicide. Convenient in use is an aerosol spray formulation in which a dye is often combined with the fungicide. The can must be held so that the spray does not come in contact with the cat's eyes, lips, or nose. This second method also minimises handling.

As a first-aid measure, tincture of iodine may be very sparingly applied to the area, if small, and especially its edges; but if the cat is to have veterinary treatment almost immediately, it is better not to apply the tincture.

As ringworm is readily transmissible to children, and less readily to adults, precautions must be taken in washing of hands after touching the cat, and with bedding material, baskets, etc. Fungal spores can survive for a very long time, but thorough vacuum cleaning will help to remove most of them in the home.

Viral Infections

Mention should be made of two viral infections of cats which give rise either to intense itching or to a burning sensation (only the cat knows which).

Rabies is one of these infections, and sometimes leads to self-mutilation; the other is **Aujeszky's disease** ('pseudo-rabies') which only rarely affects the cat. Farm cats are perhaps most likely to suffer from this disease, as it may be present (often in a subclinical form) in piggeries; it also occurs in rats.

6 Parasitic Worm Control

'My cat never has worms' is as empty a boast as 'my cat never has fleas'. True, the cat-owner may not see the worms, but they may still be there inside the animal. It is virtually impossible for any cat outside a laboratory to escape worm infestation altogether. Roundworms and tapeworms would not have continued to exist were they not successful parasites, able to ensure the survival of the species through successive generations. However, one should not be too dogmatic and suggest that all cats are infested all the time. No worms were found in 35 city cats examined *post mortem* in the Netherlands, nor in 35 per cent of unwanted and stray cats in Canberra, nor in 35 out of 110 cats in Sheffield; but it is safe to say that such a state of bliss would not have prevailed throughout their lives.

Even the most fastidious and hygiene-conscious person cannot prevent a cat becoming infested; but by periodic dosing with a prescribed anthelmintic he or she can control such infestations. It is highly desirable that this is accepted as a part of responsible cat ownership, and carried out regularly.

The word 'control' is used advisedly, because it would be misleading to imply that one dose of an anthelmintic will dispose of every worm in the cat's body. The larval stages of some worms are not affected by drugs which kill the adult worms; and so a second dose will be necessary. Again, not all anthelmintics are effective against all types of worms, so let your vet prescribe a safe and reliable one suitable for *your* cat.

Roundworms

Worms in the digestive 'tunnel' steal nourishment which should be going to the cat. Some worms cause additional harm through the secretion of toxins. Damage to the mucous membrane lining the gut may also be caused, facilitating the entry of bacteria. A massive infestation can lead to actual blockage of the intestine. On the other hand, many light infestations give rise to no observable symptoms.

Anaemia can be caused, especially by hookworms (*Ancylostoma* species) which secrete a substance inhibiting the normal clotting of the blood, for it is this upon which they feed. While infection may occur by mouth in the usual way, hookworm larvae are able to penetrate intact skin and enter the cat's body by this means.

Ascarid worms and whipworms may cause intermittent diarrhoea and vomiting, and a pot-belly in the young cat; but a harsh, lustreless coat is a more typical symptom.

Ascarid worms include *Toxocara cati* and *Toxascaris leonina*. One naturally infested cat had eight female and four male *T. cati* worms, and was passing almost 200,000 Toxocara eggs per day for 10 days.[1] The potential public health aspect of Toxocara worms is discussed in chapter 22.

The body's defence mechanism forms antibodies against parasitic worms just as it does against bacteria and viruses; and these antibodies give the adult cat a greater resistance to some worms than that possessed by kittens.

Lungworms

As might be expected, these cause coughing. In many light infestations, symptoms are so mild as to escape the cat-owner's attention; but, especially if the cat is ailing from some additional cause, the illness may be more severe, rarely fatal.

Case history. A female cat had diarrhoea and a cough for several weeks and became emaciated, weighing only 5 lb. Treatment was successful in expelling ascarid worms and reducing the diarrhoea, but then coughing increased. Live lungworm larvae were found in her faeces. A different anthelmintic was then used, and in five weeks she was well again, lungworms gone.[2]

Partly perhaps because lungworm infestation seldom causes cat-owners to seek veterinary advice, and also because of failure of older flotation test methods to demonstrate the worm eggs, this condition is only rarely recorded. However, Dr J.M. Hamilton M.R.C.V.S. found an infestation rate of over 9 per cent among 135 autopsied cats in Scotland.

Heartworms

These infest cats not only in the tropics but even in New York State. Mosquitoes and gnats transmit the minute larvae of *Dirofilaria immitis*. The adult worm lives in the right ventricle of the heart or the pulmonary artery, as a rule. If only one or two worms are present no symptoms may be shown; otherwise a cough, weakness, disinclination to play, and rapid breathing. A specific anthelmintic is necessary for treatment.

Tapeworms

In the adult cat the presence of these may be unaccompanied by obvious symptoms, but sometimes anaemia, digestive upsets, and nervous symptoms may result.

When fresh, tapeworm segments are whitish, flat, and almost rectangular, but they soon become yellowish and more like grains of rice. Gravid segments of *Dipylidium* are capable of movement.

Fleas are carriers of tapeworm larvae, and so flea control measures are necessary in addition to use of an anthelmintic effective against tapeworms.

Flukes

Like tapeworms, flukes are flat worms. In Britain the leaf-shaped liver fluke of cattle and sheep is not regarded as of any importance for the cat; but overseas the liver fluke *Platynosomum* is the cause of so-called 'lizard poisoning'. This has been reported from the U.S.A., the Caribbean islands, South America, Malaysia and Nigeria. Lizards, a large land snail, a crustacean, and amphibious creatures are hosts to various stages of the fluke's development. If numerous, the flukes can produce in the cat listlessness, fever, jaundice, diarrhoea, vomiting, and emaciation.

In North America a lung fluke, *Paragonimus*, sometimes infests cats, causing loss of weight and coughing.

REFERENCES

1 Dubey, J.P. *Vet.Rec.* 81 (1967), 671
2 Cannon, R. and Zuborg, J. *Southwestern Vet.* 19 (1966), 318

7 Two Preventable Illnesses

The importance of preventive vaccination cannot be over-emphasised when one considers the following disease: a potential killer.

Feline Infectious Enteritis (Panleukopaenia)

Caused by a virus, this illness is sudden in onset, and all too often rapidly fatal. Treatment seldom has much chance of success because there is usually insufficient time for remedial measures to take effect.

Vomiting *may* be the first symptom that the owner notices, but in typical cases what attracts attention is the cat's sudden and intense depression, with signs of abdominal pain. Often the cat prefers to lie in cold places, and may cry out. In the initial stages the temperature may rise to 105°F, or even higher, but it often becomes subnormal within 12 to 18 hours. Vomiting is quickly followed by prostration. Diarrhoea is not an invariable symptom.

Tongue ulcers may be seen in some patients; while in young kittens brain involvement may give rise to a staggering gait.

Diagnosis can be confirmed by laboratory means: the examination of blood smears which show a significantly reduced white blood cell count (panleuko-paenia). It is this which greatly reduces the cat's powers of resistance, and enables bacteria to mount an attack additional to that of the virus.

In making his diagnosis, the veterinary surgeon has to consider the possibility of poisoning, intestinal foreign bodies, and septicaemia.

Treatment is aimed at overcoming the serious dehydration which occurs in this illness. Antiserum, though expensive, may be used in a sometimes successful attempt to counter the action of the virus itself, while antibiotics may be administered to control secondary bacterial infection. Vitamins are given, and attempts made to reduce vomiting (and diarrhoea, if present). All too often, however, intensive care is of no avail, and the cat dies despite every effort to save its life; especially when treatment has been delayed.

'Prevention is better than cure' is certainly true of Feline Infectious Enteritis. It is recommended that breeding queens should be vaccinated (before mating, not during pregnancy). The kittens subsequently born will be protected by this means for the first month(s) of their lives. (For vaccination of kittens, see chapter 21.) Booster doses are advisable since immunity wanes after a time, leaving the adult cat largely unprotected.

Probably a mild form of the disease occurs in some localities at times, as many older cats have antibodies to this infection present in their blood serum, yet their owners are unable to recall any severe illness in their cats' past.

Cat Flu

'Feline influenza', or 'cat flu', is an inaccurate but convenient and widely used term for illness caused by a number of different viruses. At the time of writing, it includes **feline viral rhinotracheitis**, caused by a herpes virus, and **feline calicivirus** infection. As the two illnesses are virtually indistinguishable outside a laboratory, it is not a bad idea for them to be grouped together under a common name.

Feline viral rhinotracheitis (F.V.R.) was discovered in the U.S.A., and first recorded in Britain in the mid-1960s. In typical cases symptoms are: loss of appetite, dejection, sneezing, conjunctivitis, a discharge from the nose, and sometimes much coughing. Ulcers may form on the tongue. The cat may salivate.

This illness is seldom severe except in cats under six months old, but in them it may prove fatal. **Bronchopneumonia** is one complication which may occur, giving rise to rapid and laboured breathing, sometimes followed by exhaustion, prostration and death within a week.

Another complication which may persist after recovery in a very small proportion of patients is a chronic infection of a nasal sinus.

Treatment of F.V.R. may include the use of a steam vaporiser, fluid therapy to overcome dehydration, and antibiotics to control secondary bacterial invaders. Vitamins and baby foods may help.

Feline Calicivirus infection, the second component of 'cat flu', presents similar symptoms, though Dr R.C. Povey has stated that tongue ulcers are more common in this infection than in F.V.R., whereas coughing is less in evidence. Treatment is along similar lines.

A single 'Feline Influenza' vaccine is available for protection against both these infections and, since they can kill kittens, vaccination is well worth discussing with your veterinary surgeon. Moreover, the owners of many boarding catteries wisely refuse admission to cats for which no certificate of vaccination can be produced. This is understandable, since infection spreads rapidly from one cat to another, even if not in direct contact, through contamination of the air by virus-containing droplets emanating from sneezing cats, and from contamination of feeding bowls.

Case history. In two outbreaks of F.V.R. in a quarantine cattery, the first lasted 31 days and affected 14 out of 22 cats. The second outbreak occurred 16 weeks later, and 8 out of 16 cats became ill, two of which died. The age of the cats ranged from five months to eight years. Siamese were affected to the extent of 100 per cent and 80 per cent, respectively, in the two outbreaks; compared with 75 per cent and 50 per cent, respectively, in non-pedigree cats. None of the cats had tongue ulcers; otherwise the symptoms were as described above.[1]

Other infections which may affect the nose and/or lungs are referred to in chapter 12.

REFERENCE
1 Richmond, Philip *J. Small Anim. Pract.* 7 (1966), 451

8 Nursing an Ill Cat at Home

If your cat has an infectious disease, nursing will have to be undertaken at home, since veterinary hospitals cannot admit such cases owing to the risk to other cats. Nursing can be time-consuming, sometimes disheartening; but it can influence recovery and prove rewarding.

Nursing Practice

In nursing a cat one has to bear in mind two things: the natural recuperative powers of the body, and the will to live. The latter is important, and the cat is less likely to lose it if at home rather than in strange surroundings among strange people; to put it another way, the stress of being sent away could tip the balance.

An animal which is ill seeks solitude and requires peace. Continual fussing and interference, however well meant, are to be avoided. Good nursing implies the minimum of interference, and handling — as opposed to being with — at fairly long intervals. (This is something which has to be impressed on children. Young children should be kept away.) Fresh air, dryness, warmth, and an absence of bright lights and noise — these are points to consider when choosing a room for the cat to be in, and virtually rule out any room containing a TV set. A patient with eye inflammation, tetanus, or other illness in which nervous symptoms occur, needs protection from strong light.

Some cats seek human care and attention when they are in pain or ill; others resent any interference, sometimes to a degree which renders nursing difficult.

Two sanitary trays will be needed — perhaps three — for an ill cat confined to the house, and frequent changing of litter may be necessary as feline fastidiousness nearly always prevents re-use of already soiled litter. Old newspaper should be placed under the trays.

Drinking water should be fresh and always available. A cat with chronic nephritis needs to drink more water than it did in its younger days, for if kidney function is impaired extra water is needed to ensure elimination from the bloodstream of waste products. If vomiting is a problem, barley-water (which will be refused at first) may be tried. A cat which is losing large quantities of water and salts as a result of persistent diarrhoea urgently needs this loss making good. An injection of glucose-saline, which a veterinary surgeon will give, is the best way of achieving this. An ice cube out of a refrigerator may be offered to a cat to lick if there is haemorrhage from the stomach.

Forcible feeding exhausts and distresses an ill cat, and can do more harm

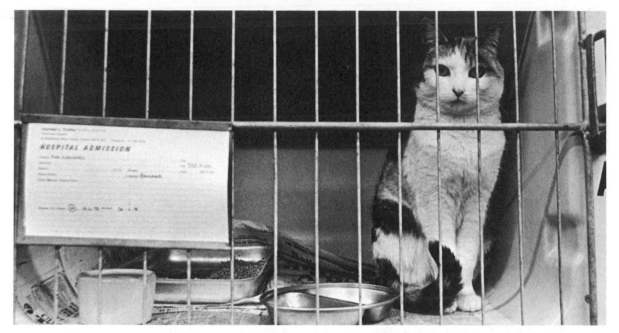

Fig 32
A patient in a
veterinary hospital.
With some infectious
diseases, the risk to
other cats makes
admission to hospital
undesirable, and so
nursing at home will
have to be undertaken.

than good; moreover, it may be violently resisted if the cat has sufficient strength. Often a short period of fasting is what the cat needs most, especially with digestive disorders.

However, since cats evidently attach much importance to the smell (as well as the taste) of their food, they may refuse to eat when suffering from a catarrhal inflammation of the nose — which causes a temporary loss of the sense of smell. In such cases, placing a single morsel of some favourite food into the cat's mouth may induce the animal to take more of its own accord. An alternative is to smear a little appetising food on to the cat's nose, from which it will be licked into the mouth, when normal feeding may be resumed.

Human invalid foods can be tried, or small pieces of rabbit or chicken, or meat jelly. Hydrolised protein is a valuable invalid food for cats, and so is glucose in milk for those unable to take solids.

Constipation is sometimes a problem. A little of the oil from a can of sardines may be taken voluntarily, whereas liquid paraffin will not. But remember that ineffectual straining of a cat over its sanitary tray may indicate difficulty in passing urine rather than faeces.

Dosing with a liquid medicine can sometimes be accomplished by the owner with the aid of a plastic eye-dropper, aimed so that its contents go on to the back of the tongue; but some cats will resist such dosing. Whether the medicine has an unpleasant taste or not, the cat *may* salivate profusely, and the medicine will then be ejected from the mouth along with the excess saliva. A subcutaneous injection of a different medicinal preparation is sometimes preferable and better tolerated.

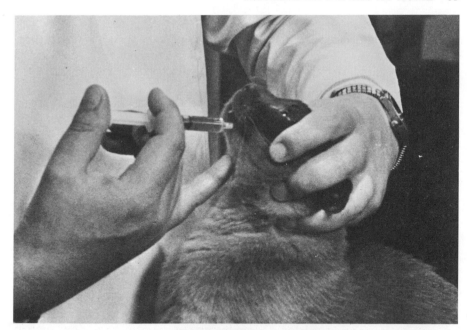

Fig 33
Giving a cat liquid
medicine by means of a
syringe.
Fig 34
Giving a cat a capsule.

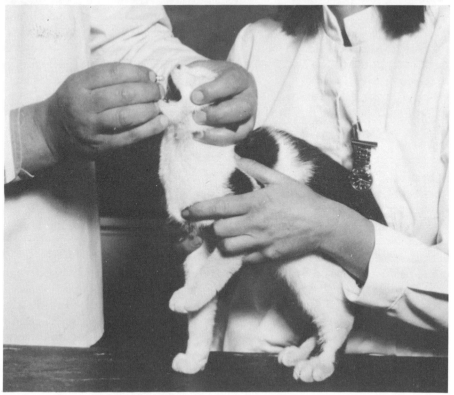

Pills are easier to give than liquids. Tablets are sometimes too large to be given this way unless broken into two or three portions, which means struggling to dose two or three times. It is better to crush a tablet and mix it into butter which can be smeared on the teeth. If the taste of the butter masks the taste of the tablet, all may be well.

Inhalations. Surprisingly, many cats are tolerant of medicated steam inhalations, should these be recommended by the veterinary surgeon. Personal experience has shown that even the strong-smelling Friar's Balsam will provoke only token resistance.

Temperature-taking is greatly resented by some cats, and it is essential to lubricate the thermometer (which should have a stubby end and not an easily broken long, thin one) adequately with Vaseline or cooking oil before insertion into the rectum. The normal temperature of a cat varies from about 101°F to 101.5°. A subnormal temperature is a danger sign.

The *pulse* can be felt on the inside of the thigh, where the femoral artery runs. A cat's pulse rate is normally between 110 and 120 times per minute.

Cleanliness. When ill, or very old, a cat may cease to perform its usual toilet; indeed, ceasing to wash itself is a sign of illness. In these circumstances, it is necessary to cut away with blunt-ended scissors any fur which has become badly soiled or matted. Diluted, warmed antiseptic solution, such as TCP, Milton, Cetrimide, or a teaspoonful of common table salt to a pint of water, can be used for washing away discharges, etc. If the nostrils become caked with discharge, most of this can be wiped away with cotton wool moistened in the saline solution mentioned above. A little olive oil can be used, if necessary, on a dry, cracked nose. If the eyelids become badly caked with discharge, relief can be afforded by bathing with saline. Boracic acid is not recommended for this purpose. Saline solution also serves as a mouth wash.

All these various procedures should be carried out very gently, but quickly, so that they do not constitute a prolonged ordeal for the cat.

Bedding. A cat which is obliged to be prostrate for long periods needs fairly soft bedding, and periodic turning over on to the other side. A lining of newspaper is useful as, if it becomes soiled, it can be removed and burnt. Freedom from draughts is, of course, essential, especially in cases of bronchitis or pneumonia, and a high-sided box, with a part cut away to provide an entrance/exit, may be acceptable.

A useful insight into some aspects of feline nursing may be obtained from the following report.

Case history. A patient with tetanus (rare in the cat) was nursed in a darkened room. A rubber mattress was used for bedding. Periodically gentle pressure was exerted on the urinary bladder. The professional treatment comprised specific anti-tetanus treatment by intravenous injection; glucose saline was given subcutaneously over a period of seven days; penicillin by intramuscular injection for five days; and, by giving promazine hydrochloride injections for 10 days, muscle relaxation was achieved, enabling the cat to swallow a small quantity of hydrolised protein an hour afterwards. The cat made a complete recovery.[1]

Middle and Old Age

In middle age many cats tend to put on weight, and some become the victims of obesity. The latter condition is one to guard against because the overweight cat is prone to various ailments less likely to affect a cat in good condition. Obesity imposes a strain on the heart and arteries, and may shorten the cat's life.

Adjust the diet of a cat which is becoming too fat. Reduce the total quantity of food slightly, and also the proportion of carbohydrate and fat. If this does not produce a slimming effect, seek veterinary advice.

In some instances obesity results from a hormone imbalance, and veterinary treatment can correct this in a majority of cases. In other instances a cat may regularly 'dine out', i.e. accept meals from two different households, and this may present a peculiarly feline problem.

Before leaving the subject of obesity it is important to emphasise that owners sometimes mistake a thin cat with *ascites* (dropsy) for a fat cat, since they judge by the pendulous abdomen, and fail to notice that the spine and ribs are poorly covered with flesh.

Elderly cats differ in their dietary needs from those of the young cat. Less fat, less carbohydrate, but adequate amounts of good-quality protein are required; with smaller meals three or four times a day.

Plenty of fresh drinking water should be available, as many elderly cats suffer from chronic nephritis and need to drink more than they used to do; and, as mentioned above, a second sanitary tray should be provided.

Decayed or loose teeth, or an accumulation of tartar, around teeth and gum edges, can cause distress and difficulty in eating, as well as giving the breath a foul odour. Tartar removal, and extraction of any loose or decayed teeth, can sometimes result in near-rejuvenation — to the surprise and delight of the owner — and undoubtedly in a happier cat.

Fainting fits may occur in an elderly cat, but the owner should not become unduly worried about these, certainly not to the extent of trying to force whisky or brandy into the reluctant animal. A short course of a suitable heart tonic may be beneficial, so ask your veterinary surgeon.

There may be disease of one of the heart valves, resulting in symptoms resembling those of human asthma, with difficulty in breathing, or a cough.

It is usually possible to alleviate, over the short term, the severity of symptoms arising from defective heart action, but not to rectify the underlying cause. Owners should take comfort from the fact that many cats with heart disease of one kind or another live to a ripe old age, and certainly do not need to be kept permanently on drugs. A heart tonic as a standby for bad periods may be all that is needed.

Some impairment of hearing and vision are to be expected in the very old cat.

Senile alopecia affects some cats. Judicious hormone treatment can sometimes correct this, so that the fur grows again over the bald patches.

Euthanasia

There may come a time when it is kinder to end a pet cat's life than to allow a miserable existence to continue. Paralysis, or an inoperable malignant growth which is causing pain, are obvious examples of circumstances warranting euthanasia.

REFERENCES
1 Miller, .E.R. *Vet.Rec.* 75 (1963), 135

9 Accidents and Other Emergencies

'Good king of cats, nothing but one of your nine lives.'
(*Romeo and Juliet*, III: i). The saying 'Cats have nine lives' contains an element of truth, in that some cats have many narrow escapes, but it should not blind us to the fact — indeed, it implies — that accidents do befall these creatures. Some of these accidents can be avoided, given a little thought by the owner.

Foreign Bodies

For example, a needle is a common foreign body in the cat, so, when you have finished your sewing, do put needles (threaded or not) away out of the cat's reach. Fishing tackle presents a hazard, too. A barbed hook caught in the tongue or swallowed is one danger, and so is the nylon or other line in which a cat may become entangled and injured.

Scalds and Burns

The kitchen can be a dangerous place for cats. Burns may result from a cat jumping on to the hotplate of an electric cooker, and I recall a horribly scalded cat; the accident occurred when a small child reached up for a saucepan on a gas cooker, drew the pan to the edge, and then accidentally tipped it over the unfortunate animal below. In the bathroom a cat may fall, or be pushed, into very hot bath water.

Scalds and burns are, of course, extremely painful, but first-aid can reduce both pain and shock if applied immediately. Hold the affected part of the cat's body under a slowly running cold tap. This will quickly reduce the temperature of the injured skin and minimise shock. Having done that, take the cat for veterinary treatment, which will probably comprise the use of pain-killers, and antibiotics to prevent serious infection.

With chemical burns, wash off the offensive material, but be careful not to spread it. For a burn caused by car-battery acid, use bicarbonate of soda in the water or, failing that, a little washing soda. Lemon juice or tannic acid may be used for a burn caused by a caustic alkali.

Electric Shock

Kittens occasionally chew the flex of an electrical appliance, causing burns in the mouth, perhaps loss of consciousness, or death. If the animal has stopped breathing, lay it on its side and apply artificial respiration by placing one hand on the chest and alternately pressing (gently) and releasing at intervals of two or three seconds.

With an apparently drowned cat, the same technique may be used, but first hold the cat head downwards and swing it to and fro a few times to clear water from the air passages.

Cats rescued from burning buildings may need artificial respiration, too, but if breathing, the vital requirement is oxygen.

Heat exhaustion implies a depletion of body fluids (dehydration) and of salts normally present in the blood. The effects may be combined with those of heat stroke, in which the ambient temperature is so high that the hypothalamus in the brain can no longer prevent body temperature from rising to a dangerously high level. For first-aid, as well as causes, see chapter 4, where hypothermia is also mentioned.

Road Accidents

A cat which has been struck a glancing blow by a motor vehicle may be in pain and seek solitude rather than return home, or may be too dazed to find its way back. If the head has been struck, there may be concussion; consciousness returning perhaps minutes, perhaps hours, after its loss. In either event, the cat may be missing, its fate unknown for a day or two. A skull fracture is likely to prove fatal; while if the spine is fractured there will be paralysis of the hind legs.

Case history 1. After a road accident a five-month-old cat kept its right foot off the ground. Veterinary examination revealed a painful swelling in the right shoulder region. X-rays showed that no fracture was present. What had occurred was separation of the muscular attachments of the scapula. A plaster-of-Paris bandage was applied across shoulder and chest, and fortunately well tolerated. After three weeks the animal was taking some weight on the leg, and after six months recovery was complete.[1]

All fractures, except a greenstick fracture in a kitten, are serious injuries, but the cat's recuperative powers plus modern veterinary surgery can achieve recovery in the majority of cases; so, apart from the two fractures mentioned above, there is no cause for initial despair on the part of the owner.

Even with fracture of the pelvis, the outlook is good provided that the cat can be closely confined for a few weeks. A remarkable escape from death was related by a fellow veterinarian, Norman Comben B.Sc, M.R.C.V.S., in his book *Dogs, Cats and People*.[2] It concerned a cat which slipped while trying to catch birds and fell from an eighth-floor window, crashed through a plate-glass roof at first-floor level, and landed in the basement. My friend, who in those days had a practice in South Kensington, treated the cat for a broken pelvis and numerous cuts. It made an excellent recovery.

Incidentally, when a fracture of the pelvis occurs in an unneutered female, she should be spayed following recovery rather than allowed to become pregnant, as there is always a very real risk of dystokia, and that would almost certainly involve a Caesarean operation.

Many limb fractures can, like those of the pelvis, be left to heal naturally, aided by either strapping or light plaster casts, again with the proviso that the cat can be kept closely confined for a period of weeks. In fractures of the humerus, femur and tibia, bone-pinning may be resorted to in order to secure apposition of the broken ends and immobilisation.

Case history 2. A bone graft was used in a remarkable and successful attempt to save the right hindleg of a Siamese which had been shot, smashing the femur and leaving several small fragments. After these had been removed, it was found impossible to use a bone plate, since there was too little of the upper femur left to provide a solid purchase with even a single screw. Accordingly, a pin was inserted into the marrow cavity of the femur, and wiring was also used. As rotation was thought likely to be a problem, notches were cut both in the Siamese's bone and in the transplant from a donor cat. After three weeks the plaster cast was removed. Fifteen months later the cat was walking normally.[3]

A plaster cast may have to be used in some fractures of the tail bones. This accident is usually caused by someone closing a door before the cat's tail is clear. Painful bruising of muscles and skin occur. Professional treatment is needed.

A fall from a height often results in a fracture of the jaw. In some instances the facial expression is altered. There is likely to be much bleeding, perhaps a broken tooth or two, bruising of the lips, with saliva perhaps dripping from the mouth, which may hang slightly open. Treatment may involve use of surgical wire to keep the fractured ends in apposition.

Traumatic cleft palate may occur at the same time as fracture of the jaw. Here again, feeding is difficult or impossible without treatment. It may be necessary to suture together the two halves of the cleft palate in order to close the gap, through which food otherwise escapes. Healing usually takes place satisfactorily.

Bleeding from the mouth may occur with the injuries just mentioned, and also when the tongue is bitten by the cat at the moment of impact during a road accident, or if the tongue is cut on the sharp lid of a food can. Haemorrhage may be alarming, and if the gash is a deep one (in the latter case), sutures may have to be inserted both to control the bleeding and hasten healing, as well as reducing subsequent pain during feeding.

A *ventral hernia* (see chapter 11) may be the sequel to an accident. Rupture of the diaphragm is, fortunately, an uncommon injury. The cat may stay in a sitting position, the breathing laboured. Haemorrhage and shock may be present to a variable degree.

Internal haemorrhage may follow a crush injury to the liver, or rarely to the

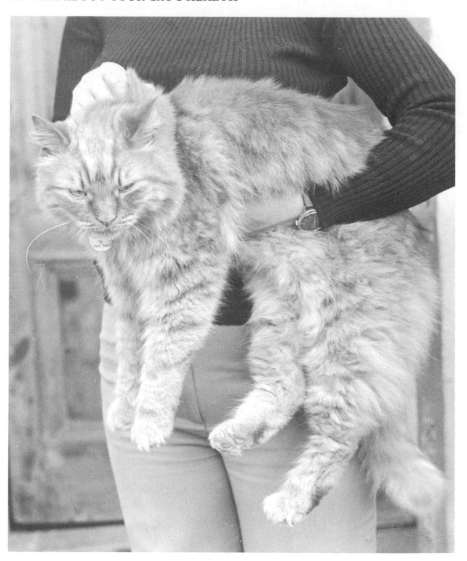

Fig 35
How to carry an
injured cat.

spleen, or to severance of any major blood vessel. Shock, characterised by an abrupt fall in blood pressure, results; breathing becomes shallow, the pulse weak, and the gums very pale indeed.

All this mention of fractures and haemorrhage may depress the reader, so let me introduce a cheerful note. In some accidents the cat has a very woebegone appearance when found dazed or frightened, with blood perhaps almost covering the face; yet, surprisingly, perhaps no lasting damage has been inflicted, and after professional treatment the cat may well present a very different picture after 48 hours — perhaps even after 24. So it is better not to abandon hope at the outset and rush off demanding euthanasia.

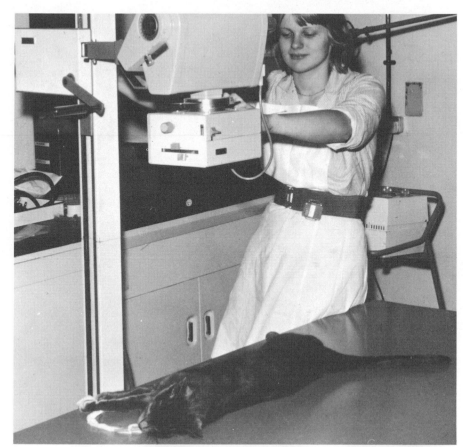

Fig 36
An anaesthetised cat awaiting radiography at the Beaumont Animal Hospital, Royal Veterinary College.
Fig 37
A bandage on a cat's leg needs to have a padding of cotton-wool underneath.

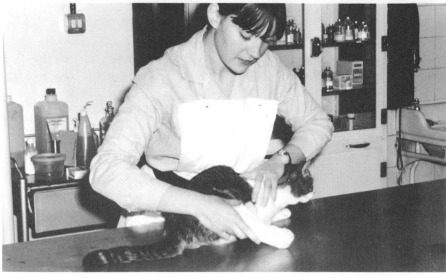

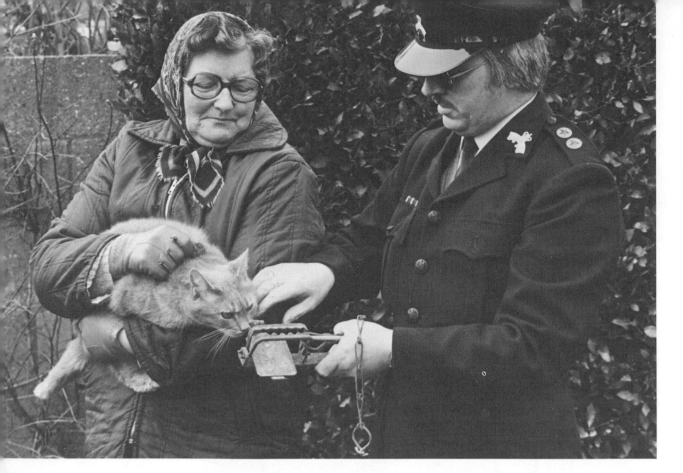

Fig 38
This cat, Sammy, now
safe in the arms of his
owner, returned home
dragging the trap
which RSPCA
Inspector John
Norman is holding.
Sammy's leg was badly
injured by the jaws of
the trap.

Dislocations

As in man, so in cats, a very wide yawn is reportedly capable of causing a
dislocated jaw. However, most dislocations are due to violence, and they may
occur concurrently with fractures.

Dislocation of the hip results in a shortening of the limb, with the foot
usually held off the ground. When the two sides of the animal are compared,
symmetry is seen to have been lost. Treatment involves reducing the dislocation under anaesthesia and then confining the cat within a small space for a
few weeks. Recovery is usually complete.

Dislocations in other regions are broadly similar in effects and treatment.

Lameness From Other Causes

Cats caught in traps or bitten by a dog, or suffering deep cuts, may become
intensely lame as a result of **severed tendons**. The ends of these can be
sutured together in some cases at least, if treated early.

Another cause or lameness is **rupture** of one or both cruciate ligaments.
These are arranged like the letter X and prevent over-extension of the stifle
joint (knee).

Injuries to the pads of the feet: (see chapter 4). Apart from slowly developing degenerative changes in a joint, **arthritis** may be due to trauma and infection; e.g. following a cat bite or dog bite. There may be severe lameness, swelling of the joint, and evidence of pain. If the joint capsule has been penetrated, there may be a sticky discharge. The danger of septicaemia is then great, but fortunately antibiotics can help here. Symptoms of illness may be seen; dejection, loss of appetite, fever.

Wounds

Fighting between rival tom cats accounts for a large proportion of feline wounds, with abscess formation as a common sequel. Dog bites, being caught in traps or snares, cuts from broken glass or the lids of food cans, and road accidents account for many more. Wounds vary, of course, from abrasions such as a graze to a deep gash extending down to the bone; from punctures made by air-gun 'slugs' or sharp-pointed objects, to lacerated wounds caused by an attacker's teeth.

Case history 3. After being missing for three days, a cat was seen to have a neck wound, and would not take food. On examination the wound was found to be a deep, infected laceration which extended through the trachea. Surgical cleaning of the wound was carried out, and the very badly damaged trachea was sutured. The cat made an excellent recovery.[4]

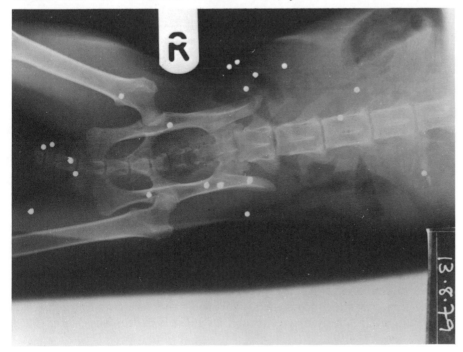

Fig 39
Lead shot widely dispersed in the body of a cat. This can result from a shooting accident but, more commonly, is the result of deliberate use of a shotgun to deter cats from gardens.

Any other type of gaping wound is also going to need stitches. This means professional help, and the sooner the better, for after several hours it may be impossible to draw the lips of the wound together, and healing will take very much longer. The only exception is a badly infected wound where there is a drainage problem.

With the exception of a cut paw, which obviously needs protection, most wounds are best left uncovered, unless the cat is constantly licking the part to an extent which inhibits healing or gives rise to a mass of 'proud flesh' or 'lick *granuloma*'. An Elizabethan collar may then be necessary.

FIRST-AID FOR WOUNDS.

The fur must be cut away with blunt-pointed scissors to allow at least ¼-inch of bare skin around the margins of the wound. The fur must not be allowed to fall into the wound and to prevent this happening, a piece of cotton-wool wrung out of warm water should be used as a temporary plug or covering for the wound — cat permitting! When the wet cotton-wool is removed, the cut fur will come away with it. Then apply normal saline (1 teaspoonful of common salt to 1 pint of warm water), or a few drops of diluted antiseptic such as Milton. (TCP and Dettol are excellent, too, but the strong smell of these may worry the cat.) Boracic acid is likely to be worse than useless.

A clean, healthy wound is pink. Any yellowish-green scab must always be removed and not mistaken for a healed surface. The wound must heal from below upwards. If a scab is left on top, healing will be delayed since pus is likely to accumulate below it.

Sometimes a wound may ulcerate, with raised edges and a tough, adherent greenish-yellow base. Professional help will usually be needed, as ulcers are very resistant to ordinary home treatment.

Other Emergencies

Some of these are dealt with in chapter 15; for example, where a sudden swelling of the abdomen occurs, or the cat is showing signs of pain, or vomiting. Unsuccessful attempts to pass urine, with a full bladder and pain when the abdomen is gently pressed, is certainly an emergency.

If, during the summer, a cat has come in from the garden showing profuse salivation, retching, vomiting, or subsequent loss of consciousness, it may have taken a toad into its mouth. The toad has no means of defence other than its venom, which is secreted by glands in its skin. The venom of British toads is less potent than that of some species found overseas, but it does cause severe inflammation of the mucous membrane lining the mouth and pharynx. The salivation and retching may continue, Dr P.G.C. Bedford has stated, for as long as 8 or 12 hours.

It is only very occasionally, it seems, that a cat actually swallows a toad, but if this happens symptoms of 'acute abdominal pain and continuous exhaustive vomiting' are produced after 24 hours or so. A staggering gait may be observed, or the cat may remain lying down with a fixed stare.

There are no records of adult cats in Britain dying from toad venom, but one three-month-old Persian kitten died within three days.[5]

Cats are very rarely, so far as is known, bitten by adders in this country, but overseas the situation is different. In Australia, for example, snake bite was diagnosed at the University of Melbourne in 41 cats over a six-year period; the Tiger Snake having been positively identified in seven of these cases. Symptoms included generalised weakness, dilated pupils and absence of normal reaction to light by the pupils, with vomiting and laboured breathing in some instances. The outlook is bad if there is paralysis, and a subnormal temperature. A high recovery rate followed in bitten cats receiving adequate doses (3000 units) of Tiger Snake antivenin.[6]

For **paralysis**, see chapter 17; and for a personal **rabies** emergency, chapter 23.

REFERENCES
1 Schneck, G.W. *Feline Practice* 5 (1975), 49
2 Comben, Norman. *Dogs, Cats and People* (Thames & Hudson, 1955)
3 Hendrikson, Peter. *J.Amer.Vet.Med.Assoc.* 174 (1979), 827
4 Reeder, P.L. *Vet. Record* 95 (1974), 473
5 Bedford, P.G.C. *Vet.Record* 94 (1974), 613
6 Hill, F.W.G. and Campbell, T. *Austr.Vet.J.* 54 (1978), 437

10 Accidental Poisoning

The purpose of this chapter is to indicate those circumstances in which poisoning of cats commonly occurs so that, forewarned, the owner may be able to take at least some precautions.

If the poison is known to be a chemical compound with either a proprietary name, or a long, barely pronounceable one given on the label of a packet, can or bottle, take it or the label to your veterinary surgeon, or jot down the name of the proprietary product and of the manufacturer.

In many instances, however, there will be no certainty that the cat has been poisoned; merely a strong suspicion. Diagnosis is all-important, since the symptoms of some illnesses are the same as those of some cases of poisoning, and *vice versa*. For example, not only vomiting and diarrhoea but also a high temperature, rapid breathing, excitement sometimes amounting to frenzy, convulsions, salivation, and jaundice are common to both. (Feline Infectious Enteritis outbreaks have led to 'mass poisoning' scares.)

In the Home

FOOD

As mentioned in chapter 2, meat sold in slab form as a pet food sometimes has **benzoic acid** added as a preservative. If too much is added, or if it is badly mixed so that some parts of the slab contain an excessive amount, poisoning may result. Salivation, extreme aggressiveness or frenzy, and convulsions are seen in benzoic acid poisoning, which is often fatal. One curious symptom is that the cat jumps backwards and strikes out with the fore-paws as though 'catching imaginary mice'. The frenzy associated with benzoic acid poisoning might well be mistaken for the furious form of rabies and, in countries where that disease occurs, a differential diagnosis would be called for by the attending veterinarian.

Another example of poisoning which occasionally arises from the feeding of cats not on butcher's meat but knacker's meat is that caused by **barbiturates**. When a farm animal — horse, cow, sheep or goat — has to be 'put down', a humane and convenient way of doing so is to use an overdose of a barbiturate anaesthetic given by injection. Residues of the barbiturate in the carcase may then poison a cat fed on meat from it. In one instance a cat ate a kidney from a calf killed in this way and, as a result, became unsteady on its legs, then comatose and later, when it recovered consciousness, extremely excitable.

Chloral hydrate poisoning may similarly occur in small animals fed on meat from the carcase of a farm animal humanely 'put down' with this drug.

In the 1960s an outbreak of poisoning followed the finding of a dead pony by the roadside. The dead animal was removed to a knacker's yard, whence the meat reached (through the usual trade channels) the owners of cats and dogs, of which about 100 died from **fluoroacetamide** poisoning, from which the pony itself had died. However, this was a rare and isolated case, and it would be alarmist to imply otherwise.

In Japan, some years ago, veterinary investigation established the cause of illness in cats showing nervous symptoms as **chronic mercury** poisoning. This finding solved the mystery of a similar illness, with many fatalities, in people living in the same area. Both cats and people had been poisoned through eating locally caught fish with a high mercury content as a result of industrial pollution. Similar poisoning in cats which had eaten fish caught in Moreton Bay, Tasmania, was reported by Dr T.A. Gruber and colleagues in 1978; the symptoms including loss of appetite, loss of weight, fine muscular tremors, blindness, a staggering gait, and convulsions.

For a vitamin deficiency resulting from the feeding of **raw fish**, see chapter 17.

(So-called 'food poisoning', caused by Salmonella organisms, coliform and other bacteria, is referred to in chapters 14 and 15.)

MEDICINES

It has to be said that sometimes people unintentionally poison their cats through overdosing with medicines or giving unsuitable ones. In this connection, advice from neighbours, however well-meaning and reputedly 'good with animals' they may be, should be treated with the utmost caution. For example, pay no heed to anyone recommending Easton's Syrup for cats, as this tonic contains strychnine, to which cats are extremely susceptible: a safe human dose proves lethal to them.

Cats are also highly susceptible to poisoning by **aspirin** (acetyl-salicylic acid) and **sodium salicylate**. The presentday equivalent of the old five-grain tablet (0.3 gramme) has proved fatal as a daily dose to cats over a 12-day period; and one cat died after being given 9 grains (0.58 gramme) of aspirin over a 2½-day period. Smaller doses may still make the cat ill, so these popular household remedies, as well as the banned **phenacetin**, are best not given to a cat by its owner at all. The same applies to **paracetamol**, another widely used pain-reliever which is chemically related to phenacetin, and with which an owner inadvertently poisoned her cat.

Symptoms of aspirin poisoning include salivation, vomiting, and an unsteady gait. Kittens are probably less often poisoned than are puppies through eating pills, tablets, or capsules left lying about in the home, but the risk is there, and children may give them to a cat.

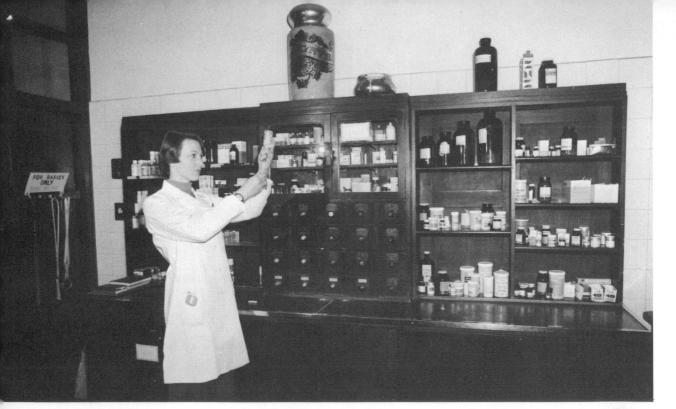

Fig 40
Inside a pharmacy at
the Royal Veterinary
College, University of
London. Of course,
medicines in the home
are stored on a rather
different scale, but the
same principles of well
organised storage
should apply. Be
careful to keep human
medicines well
separated from those
intended for cats. What
is safe for one is not
necessarily safe for the
other.

SKIN DRESSINGS

Their habit of washing themselves makes cats especially susceptible to
poisonous substances applied to their fur, or contaminating the pads of their
feet, since much of the noxious material will inevitably be swallowed. 'This
explains', commented the late Dr E.G.C. Clarke, 'why a cat is poisoned much
more readily than a dog if its coat is dusted with a flea powder containing
BHC or **DDT**, and is at much greater risk if it walks over wet **creosote**.'

Kittens, incidentally, have been poisoned when suckled by their DDT-
treated mother, since a high proportion of the insecticide is excreted from the
body via the milk. Apart from being licked, both BHC and DDT can be
absorbed through the unbroken skin of a cat being given a wet shampoo.[1]

Case history 1. A long-haired Persian cat, with notoedric mange affecting
many parts of its body, was given a preliminary bath in warm, soapy water,
and then with a suspension of BHC. Drying with a towel was carried out after
both baths, after which the cat was put out in the sun. Although no licking
was observed, symptoms appeared four hours later: shivering, mewing,
convulsions; and the animal died despite all attempts to save its life.

Another cat, treated with the BHC suspension (at the same strength) but
without the preliminary bath with soapy water, showed no ill effects; but
when the animal was treated again a week later, *after* the preliminary bath,
symptoms appeared five hours later; notably, frenzy, salivation, and later
somnolence, with recovery after a further hour. (It was suggested at the
University of Sydney that the preliminary bath possibly removed skin fat and
facilitated absorption of the BHC.[2])

Benzyl benzoate, an acaricide (mite killer) used in the treatment of mange, is also readily absorbed through the unbroken skin, and must be used with great caution on cats, or not at all. Symptoms of poisoning include great excitability; sometimes vomiting and diarrhoea as well.

Tincture of iodine is not recommended for cats, and if used at all should be confined to a single application to a very small area of skin.

Phenol (carbolic acid) and its various compounds, and **cresols**, provide other examples of poisons readily absorbed through the unbroken skin. They should never be used on cats, which are notoriously susceptible to this type of poisoning. The reason for this is, as Prof. Clarke explained at a BSAVA Congress, that the cat lacks a particular enzyme which most other animals have, and so 'has to detoxicate phenol compounds by a slower and less efficient process'.

Oil of lavender, turpentine, and **mercury** preparations are all potentially dangerous and have no place in modern feline medicine or first-aid. Turpentine should *not* be used for removing paint from cats' fur.

Case history 2. This illustrates the risk of children playing with medicines or toilet preparations and putting them on cats. A kitten became deeply unconscious after licking a baby-toilet powder containing benzalkonium chloride 'liberally applied to its fur'. [3]

Toys

These must be choosen judiciously, and plastic ones avoided.

Case history 3. A Siamese cat became unwell after playing with a plastic snake (of the kind which quivers when held in the hand or moved). She appeared to have difficulty in finding her food, and was unsteady on her legs. Later she was twitching continuously, and any sound or touch sent her into convulsions. Veterinary treatment included a drug to control these. Next day she was much less excitable, but had a temperature of 105°F. Both urine and breath had a very strong 'plasticky' smell, and during the night pieces of plastic had been vomited. (It was only then that her owner associated the poisoning with the plastic snake.) After five days of careful treatment, the cat made a complete recovery. [4]

Fumes

Many an owner has come downstairs in the morning to find the cat dead from **asphyxia**. This may occur where there is a solid fuel stove if ventilation is inadequate, or with a gas-stove.

Dr G.S. Venables, writing in *The Lancet* on the dangers of human poisoning by carbon monoxide, mentioned the content of this in various gases. In Britain, until the late 1960s, town (coal-) gas contained 10 to 20 per cent carbon monoxide. Natural and oil-based gases contain less than 1 per cent. Natural gas normally burns leaving carbon dioxide and water, but with 'inadequate ventilation and poor escape for exhaust gases, incomplete combustion to carbon monoxide may occur'. The lethal gas then accumulates rapidly and, in man, 'a 1-per-cent concentration in the atmosphere may result in 70 per cent saturation of haemoglobin, a level which may prove fatal'.

Case history 4. Two cats and a dog were found unconscious in the kitchen one morning, and there was a strong smell of gas. It was presumed that one of the cats had jumped on to the cooker and turned on one of the taps. All three animals revived when taken into fresh air, but next day all were deaf. The cats regained partial hearing in 10 days, and seemed normal 21 days after the incident.[5]

Temporary **blindness** has also been reported in cats poisoned by coal-gas.

Animals have been fatally poisoned after being left in a kitchen with a smoking chip pan.

OTHER SOURCES

In rooms which are being redecorated, cats may lick spilt **paint**, or paint scrapings, or old flaking paintwork. Red lead left behind by a plumber is another hazard. Symptoms of acute **lead poisoning** include salivation, vomiting, signs of abdominal pain, excitement, blindness, and convulsions. (A blue line around the gums is a sign of chronic lead poisoning, such as might arise in some districts where local water supplies contain traces of lead as a result of industrial pollution, but the risks of this occurring are very slight indeed. However, it is better not to offer your cat grass cut from the verge of a busy road where lead from car exhausts contaminates herbage.) Putty, linoleum, golf balls, and lead shot are other sources.

Some **house plants** are poisonous and may be nibbled by kittens with fatal results.

In the Garage

There have been many cases of puppies gaining access to car battery acid, and this could happen with kittens, too. A far more common source of poisoning in the garage is **ethylene glycol** (anti-freeze), which has a sweetish taste which cats evidently find palatable. Many cats die from this cause every year. Symptoms of ethylene glycol poisoning include depression, a staggering gait, convulsions, and coma.

In the Garden

Some cats like the taste of anti-slug pellets containing **metaldehyde** or a related compound, **methiocarb**, and eat them readily. Since successful gardening and slugs are incompatible, and if no hedgehog is resident, the best course is to continue using the pellets but to fix a piece of wire-netting (or an inverted flower-pot weighted down with a stone) over the soil where they have been placed.

Metaldehyde poisoning gives rise to convulsions, often preceded by muscular twitching, excitement and vomiting. The animal shows an exaggerated response (hyperaesthesia) to stimuli such as touch, noise, and bright light; it should therefore be kept quiet in semi-darkness until veterinary aid can be obtained. An unusual sequel to metaldehyde poisoning has been reported; namely, blindness, which gradually disappears after three weeks.

Garden hazards apply even more to the potting shed, where slug pellets may be spilt from their carton on to the floor, and where other poisons abound; for example, **nicotine**, which is readily absorbed through the unbroken skin; moss-killers; insecticides; herbicides.

Case history 5. A Siamese cat was noticed eating grass from a lawn, the weedy parts of which had been 'spot-treated' by the owner with undiluted Gramoxone (20 per cent paraquat). The cat became noticeably ill 18 hours later, being very depressed and vomiting. Taken to a veterinary hospital five hours later, the cat (quiet but alert) was kept in for observation and treatment. On the third day, loss of appetite, salivation and ulceration of the tongue were observed. Treatment included physiological saline injections, as the cat was taking no food, and this continued for 10 days. Appetite then returned, and after 15 days the cat was sent home. After a further 15 days, however, the cat was back, this time on account of loss of appetite and distressed breathing. In view of the cat's dehydrated state, fluid therapy was resumed. After a fortnight the cat was well enough to be sent home where, six months later it was breathing more rapidly than normal (presumably indicating some degree of permanent lung damage) but was 'otherwise well'.[6] Less fortunate was the same owner's fox-terrier, which died from paraquat poisoning within days of the lawn being treated.

Paraquat causes **oedema of the lungs,** and the victim 'drowns' from its own inflammatory effusions into the air-cells. This herbicide is sometimes applied by local authority workmen to roadside verges as an economical method of controlling rank growth; it is widely used by farmers; and occasionally it is illicitly used in sheep carcases as a poison bait intended to kill foxes.

Beyond the Garden

The hunting cat may, in your garden or beyond its confines, encounter a toad, and if unwise enough to take the creature into his mouth, become ill from the effects of the toad's defensive venom, called *bufotalin*. For further information on this, see chapter 9, where snake venom is also referred to.

A far greater risk attaches to the **eating of birds** poisoned by **farm**

chemicals, and the more easily caught by the cat for that reason. *Organochlorine* compounds, widely used on farms as insecticides, include BHC, aldrin, dieldrin, endrin, toxaphene and many others. Symptoms of this type of poisoning vary but, generally speaking, excitement (which may amount to aggressiveness), salivation, a staggering gait, aimless wandering, a raised body temperature, and convulsions are seen, though not all in the same animal.

Another large group of farm chemicals are the *organophosphorous* compounds, which include dichlorvos, schradan, parathion, dimefox and malathion. Poisoning by them may give rise to loss of appetite, abdominal pain, salivation, vomiting and diarrhoea, rapid breathing, convulsions, and paralysis, or to some of these symptoms.

Mercury compounds used for seed dressings sometimes poison birds and so, indirectly, cats. Dressed seed corn has been used in the manufacture of dog biscuits or meal, causing dieldrin poisoning. A similar risk applies to cats.

Strychnine is a poison commonly used against moles and, illicitly, sometimes against foxes. In my own practice I treated a dog poisoned with this within days of a rumour that pieces of poisoned sausage had been put down as bait by local council workmen to destroy rats. Cats are similarly at risk from this violent poison, which — perhaps after some excitement and muscular twitching — produces convulsions, hyperaesthesia, and opisthotonus (arching of the spine like a bow). Vomiting occasionally occurs.

Alphachloralose is used against both wood-pigeons and mice, and the risk to cats comes from eating poisoned pigeons or other birds. Symptoms include a staggering gait and, later, coma.

Warfarin is one of a group of compounds which are all anticoagulants, and kill rats and mice by inhibiting normal clotting of the blood. Another poison in this group is *cumachlor*. Cats are less likely than dogs to eat poisoned bait, but they may eat poisoned rodents, or food contaminated by rats' urine. Certainly cats are not exempt from this type of poisoning, and in a Swiss survey of 46 cases in dogs and cats, five cats became ill and two died despite treatment with vitamin K. Symptoms include anaemia, apathy, weakness, loss of appetite, a suggestion of cramp, internal haemorrhage, and sometimes subcutaneous swelling caused by bleeding. Warfarin-poisoned cats must be handled very gently, because the slightest knock may increase bleeding.

The laying of poisoned baits above ground for the destruction of rats and mice is illegal in Britain, but the law is frequently broken; as it sometimes is, no doubt, in the use of certain poisons banned under the Animals (Cruel Poisons) Act 1962. In view of this, and as such a ban does not operate in all countries, it seems worth listing the following rodenticides.

Antu. This is an abbreviation for alphanaphylthiourea, sometimes referred to as thiourea, an effective rat-killer. It causes vomiting and diarrhoea, with death from oedema of the lungs.

Barium salts (usually barium chloride) cause salivation and convulsions.

Sodium monofluoro-acetate (1080) causes pain, vomiting, and convulsions.

Yellow phosphorus, used in non-safety matches and rat poisons, produces great thirst, severe abdominal pain, vomiting, diarrhoea, and great dejection. Vomited material may be greenish in colour and luminous in the dark. *Zinc phosphide* poisoning is characterised by similar symptoms.

Red squill, prepared from the sea onion, has an unpleasant taste and odour, and fortunately baits made with this are unlikely to be eaten by cats as a rule; and when they eat rats poisoned by red squill they usually avoid eating the digestive organs. Symptoms resemble those of the organophosphorous compounds.

Thallium salts, used as rat poisons, may cause vomiting, diarrhoea, and fever, with later salivation and conjunctivitis. In less acute cases, a brick-red discoloration of the skin, and some loss of fur, are characteristic. Thallium poisoning is almost invariably fatal.

In the Cattery

While it is highly desirable to exercise efficient rodent control in and around premises where cats are bred and boarded, in view of rodent-borne diseases and possible contamination of stored cat foods by urine and faeces, care must obviously be taken in the choice and placing of poison baits.

A choice of bedding is important, too. For example, sawdust from timber treated with the wood-preservative pentachlorophenol, has proved fatal to cats. (Shavings of the red African hardwood *Mansonia altissma* have fatally poisoned dogs bedded on them, and the likelihood is that they would be similarly dangerous to cats.)

First-Aid for Poisoning

In suggesting simple first-aid measures, it must be emphasised that they necessarily differ from — and are likely to be less effective than — those measures which the veterinary surgeon will take. Accordingly, the sooner that veterinary treatment is obtained, the greater the chance of saving the cat's life.

Where poison is known to have been given by accident, or taken, an emetic is useful in most cases; for first-aid purposes, a crystal of washing soda, mustard and water, or salt and water may be given. In a cat which is already vomiting, do not further distress the animal by forcing an emetic into it.

Strong tea is useful, owing to its tannic acid content, as a first-aid antidote to strychnine and other alkaloid poisoning; and in cases of lead and zinc poisoning.

White of egg in milk is of some value also for lead and zinc poisoning, and for phenol (carbolic acid) compounds, Lysol, and corrosives.

86 ALL ABOUT YOUR CAT'S HEALTH

Vinegar or lemon juice is appropriate in poisoning by alkalis.

Milk of Magnesia or bicarbonate of soda (NOT washing soda) may be used in poisoning by an acid.

REFERENCES

1 Guilhon, J. *Proc. 15th Int.Vet.Congress,* 1953.

2 Blood, D.C. *et al. Austr.Vet.J.* 24 (1948), 131

3 *Garner's Veterinary Toxicology* (Baillière, Tyndall)

4 Stewart, J.D. and North, D.C. *Vet.Record* 100 (1977), 146

5 Comben, Norman. *Vet.Record* 61 (1949), 128

6 Johnson, R.P. and Huxtable, C.R. *Vet.Record* 98 (1976), 189

11 Lumps and Swellings

'It's this lump that I'm worried about,' a cat-owner may say in the consulting room. Very often that word 'lump' is an apt description and could not be bettered. The nature of the 'lump' is something for the veterinary surgeon to ascertain.

Haematoma

In the cat it is not at all uncommon for a swelling to appear on the inner surface of the projecting part of the ear (pinna). Such a swelling, below the skin, is usually found to be a haematoma, which contains blood or blood-clot, and may result from damage to a small blood vessel by another cat's claws during a fight. As would be expected, the entire (unneutered) tom cat's risk of having a haematoma is far greater than that of a neutered animal, simply because his life-style involves numerous battles.

However, ear mange results in much scratching, and in the process a cat may injure its own ear, with bleeding below the skin, and the appearance of this unsightly 'lump'.

The condition is not painful to the same extent as an abscess, but there will probably be both tenderness and discomfort.

Is any treatment necessary? Strictly speaking, I suppose the answer is 'No', because, unless a cat with ear mange punctures the swelling with a claw and converts the haematoma into an abscess, the blood and serum inside will gradually become absorbed. Unfortunately, this is accompanied by crinkling of the ear which is rather unsightly and results in a permanent deformity or blemish. Surgical treatment can minimise the crinkling and subsequent deformity, as well as relieving the cat of immediate and persistent discomfort.

A haematoma may, of course, occur on parts of the body other than the ear. For example, if a cat is struck by a car (or by someone wielding a stick) there will be bruising and some bleeding below the skin, giving rise to one or more swellings of the kind already described. Naturally such areas will be very tender; but no treatment of the haematoma itself is called for.

As mentioned in chapter 10, a cat which has been poisoned by warfarin (the rodenticide which inhibits clotting of the blood and so leads to death from internal haemorrhages) may show several swellings below the skin, due to bleeding occasioned by minor knocks and the failure of the bleeding to cease owing to natural clotting. Such a cat must be handled very gently, and urgently needs vitamin K treatment, etc.

Fig 41
The swelling on the
ear is a haematoma.
Fig 42
An abscess at the side
of the face due to a cat
bite.

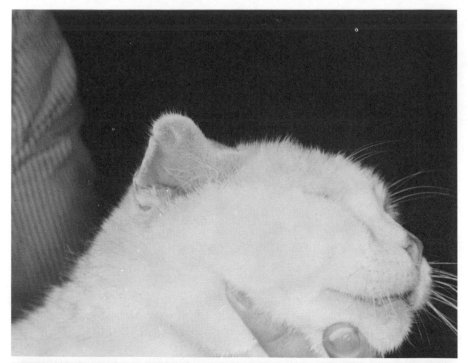

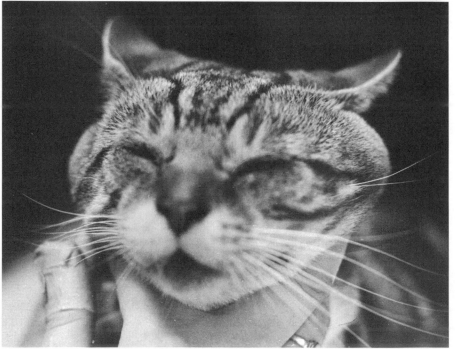

Abscess

Far more common than a haematoma is an abscess. This may occur anywhere in the body, but the swellings which you will see will obviously be just below the skin. Being bitten by a dog or another cat; penetration of a thorn, or of a grass seed; an injury from barbed wire — these are all common causes: bacteria such as streptococci and staphylococci enter through the breach in the skin and start to multiply.

Abscesses in cats are not always very typical; even the acute ones, instead of being circumscribed, are often diffuse. In other words, the infection is by no means as localised as you might expect; and many abscesses in cats do not 'point'. So the question arises: *is* it an abscess? If the swelling follows the return home of a tom cat which has obviously been involved in a fight, you may be fairly certain that abscess it is. In other cases there may be doubt — so obtain a diagnosis.

The second question which arises is whether your cat is sufficiently amenable for you to undertake first-aid, or whether you would prefer to have professional treatment from the outset.

First-aid involves hot fomentations. These reduce the pain and provide some help towards overcoming the infection, though this is more effectively tackled by antibiotics, probably essential in the end.

The simple technique of hot fomentations for a cat is similar to that for a person. Merely soak a large pad of cotton-wool, or a piece of an old sheet, in hot water, wring out most of the water, and apply to the abscess area. (The temperature should not be higher than can comfortably be borne by the point of one's elbow.) Fomentations are continued for several minutes in this way, and can be repeated three or four times a day — if the cat will accept them.

For an abscess which has burst, first-aid consists in irrigating or syringing the cavity with normal saline (one teaspoonful of kitchen salt to a pint of warm water), or with a diluted and warmed antiseptic solution, e.g. Milton, TCP, hydrogen peroxide. Then the cavity must be kept open and unbandaged. There will be a tendency for the discharge to form a scab over the opening, leading the unwary cat-owner to think that healing has occurred; but healing must take place from the bottom. If the skin joins across the top while a focus of infection remains below, the abscess will persist or recur.

Clipping of some fur around the site is essential, as otherwise it becomes matted with discharge, and the situation worse rather than better.

Accidents

If the cat has a small wound which does not heal, but continues to discharge pus, a **fistula** or **sinus** may be present (see under facial swellings, chapter 3). Veterinary attention will be needed.

Gas gangrene is very rare in the cat. Perhaps only one owner in a million will ever encounter it. There is a swelling like that of an ordinary, acute abscess, but the skin may crackle when touched, and any escaping pus will be frothy, due to gas formed by certain bacteria which have gained entrance to the tissues following a compound fracture or a deep puncture wound. Professional treatment is needed very urgently; if not forthcoming, the cat is likely to die from septicaemia. Do not waste time on first-aid measures which will be ineffective.

Hernia

A cold, painless swelling at a kitten's navel is likely to be a hernia or 'rupture'. Gentle pressure with the fingers will usually cause it momentarily to disappear. The opening in the abdominal wall is a natural one which, however, should have closed at birth. If allowed time, it may still do so. Only a persistent or irreducible **umbilical hernia** will need surgical intervention, owing to risk of a piece of omentum having its blood supply interfered with, or a piece of intestine becoming obstructed or strangulated — both serious conditions requiring surgery without delay. (Umbilical hernia is far less common in the kitten than in the puppy.)

A **ventral hernia** is usually the result of violence of some kind, resulting in a breach in the supporting muscles of the abdomen. Intestine may protrude through this unnatural opening in the muscles and be supported only by the skin. The cat's owner will notice a swelling on one side. Owing to the violence, the area may be very painful; but even if not, professional help is needed. The gap in the muscle must be closed.

Hernia may occur in other situations, but only rarely in the cat.

Ticks

An engorged tick, with its legs concealed under its bloated body, hardly looks like a parasite to anyone seeing it for the first time, and may be mistaken for a small tumour, or just another 'lump'.

Enlarged lymph nodes

Very small 'lumps' which can be felt but not seen may be lymph nodes if present in much the same situations as in human beings. When nodes are enlarged, the owner may become aware of them (see chapter 18).

Tuberculosis

Flat, sometimes oval, 'lumps' on the skin's surface may be the result of tuberculosis, and veterinary advice should be sought if these appear; the more urgently so if they are beginning to ulcerate. This cause of 'lump' is, fortunately, a rarity nowadays in cats in Britain.

Tumours

'Growths' or tumours vary greatly in appearance, rate of growth, type, and importance. Tumours on stalks are known as **polyps**. Occasionally they are found in cats' ears or in the vagina, for example.

Hollow tumours containing fluid are known as **cysts**. A 'retention cyst' may appear anywhere on the skin, and has to be distinguished from an abscess. There is no associated pain or redness (unless the swelling has been caught by the teeth of a comb during grooming), and it forms slowly. It is not at all a serious condition, and is due merely to blockage of the duct of one of the sebaceous glands which lubricate the hairs of the coat. Such a cyst often needs opening, and its contents evacuating; but not always. If it is left, be careful not to jab it with a comb.

Warts are small, solid tumours, and may have a flat top, a cauliflower-shaped top, or be irregular in shape (like human warts, in fact). They usually grow to a small size, and then do not become any bigger, and may be present for years without causing pain or discomfort. They may disappear spontaneously after a while. If a wart begins to bleed, ulcerate, or have an offensive odour — or if a large number appear in the mouth, for example — veterinary advice should be sought.

A simple **fibroma** is another type of benign tumour not uncommon in cats, and is so called on account of being composed largely of fibrous tissue. Its removal may or may not be advisable, depending on situation, and on any tendency to ulcerate.

Benign tumours grow slowly, press neighbouring parts aside, but neither invade nor destroy them (though pressure may have an adverse effect on adjacent tissues and organs). Unlike a malignant, or cancerous growth, a benign tumour does not spread to distant tissues and, once removed surgically, seldom recurs. Some do not need to be removed at all.

MALIGNANT TUMOURS

Owners sometimes express surprise when informed that cats are subject to cancer, but unfortunately they are, though to a slightly less extent than dogs.

As readers know, malignant tumours differ from benign ones in that they are, as a rule, faster growing; and they invade and destroy normal tissues, and frequently give rise to metastases (or secondary growths) in other parts of the body. Unlike a benign tumour, a cancerous growth is commonly of irregular shape and its margins are indeterminate. Separation of such a growth from the organ it has invaded may be impossible, so that the whole organ may have

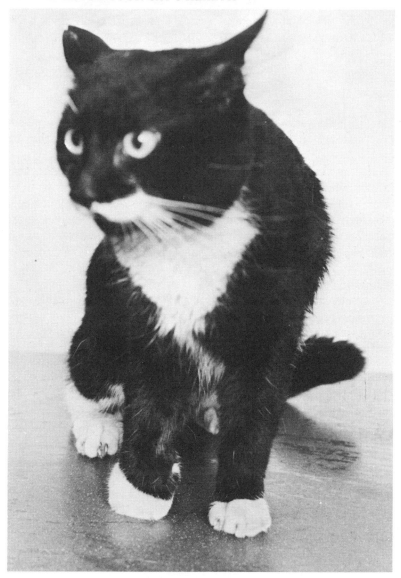

Fig 43
A swollen paw due to a
bee sting.

to be removed where that is practicable.

An example of a malignant tumour is a **fibrosarcoma** — a malignant version of the simple fibroma mentioned above: a form of skin cancer.

Surveys by veterinary pathologists in many countries have shown that the most common malignant growth in cats is a **lymphosarcoma,** but this only rarely affects the skin. In older cats a swelling affecting one or more of the mammary glands is likely to be malignant, and there is often spread to other organs and tissues.

Other Causes

LEG SWELLINGS

A painful or tender swelling of a fore- or hind-leg may be due to a malignant growth affecting the bone.

Sometimes the cause of a leg swelling *not* involving the bone is constriction of the local circulation by a rubber band placed on the leg by a child. Such a swelling is slow in onset, unlike the very rapid swelling caused by snake bite (see chapter 9). The rubber band will be so embedded that the owner will not be able to see it in most cases. Gangrene of the leg is likely to occur if the band is not found and removed by a veterinary surgeon.

A leg swelling may also be due to some other circulation defect or to infection.

SWELLING OF THE ABDOMEN

This chapter is concerned mainly with external swellings or 'lumps' appearing on the surface of the body, but a passing reference should be made here to an enlargement of the whole abdomen. Apart from pregnancy, ascites (dropsy), pyometra, or torsion of the stomach, an overfull bladder, such an enlargement may, of course, be due to the presence of an internal tumour, either benign or malignant.

12 Coughs and Sneezes

Sneezes

'Coughs and sneezes spread diseases' runs the jingle, which is true of cats as well as of human beings; and the sounds are enough to induce alarm or despondency in the owners of quarantine, boarding, or breeding catteries. An outbreak of '**cat flu**' is described in chapter 7.

Another infection of the upper air passages is **Feline pneumonitis**, which is accompanied by similar but milder symptoms, similar to those of the common cold in man. Sneezing is a feature of both these viral infections.

The viruses attack the mucous membrane lining the air passages, giving rise to a catarrhal inflammation. The result is that extra mucus is produced by the membrane's goblet cells which, in health, secrete mucus for purposes of lubrication. The 'extra' mucus in catarrh forms the watery discharge with which we are all personally familiar. Later the discharge thickens and may become greenish-yellow. The term 'muco-purulent' is applied to it, since it now consists not merely of mucus but also of tissue débris, live and dead defensive white blood cells, virus, and bacteria — the secondary invaders which were enabled to take advantage of the inflammation caused by the virus. Irritation of the nerve endings causes sneezing.

If much muco-purulent discharge is present, coughing — another reflex action — may be induced in order to clear the airways.

Although viral infections are the most common cause of sneezing, this may also occur in cases of allergy of the hay-fever type or if there is a grass seed lodged in the nose.

A muco-purulent discharge from one nostril only may indicate the presence of a foreign body or a **fungal infection** of nose or nasal sinus. Fungal infection may occur where the nasal sinus is already the site of a tumour.

Case history 1. A spayed two-year-old cat had been snuffling for some time when an ulcer appeared at the right nostril. A week later a second ulcer appeared below the right eye, and a whitish 'lump' protruded from it. Breathing now became noisy, and from the right nostril came a muco-purulent discharge. Yeast-like bodies were found and identified, by laboratory means, as Cryptococcus. The cat was 'put down'.[1]

Coughs

Coughing may be a symptom not only of the viral infections already mentioned, but of many other conditions.

Case history 2. The sudden onset of coughing, with gulping or retching, in three different cats, was found under anaesthesia to be due to blades of grass or grass seeds caught in the pharynx and above the soft palate.[2]

Tonsillitis is not common in cats, but when it does occur it can give rise to coughing as well as retching or difficulty in swallowing.

Case history 3. A 10-month-old cat had been vomiting occasionally and evinced difficulty in swallowing. There were ulcers on both of the enlarged and protruding tonsils (normally concealed from view in their crypts). Antibiotics failed to control Pasteurella and Moraxella organisms isolated from throat swabs, but complete recovery followed tonsillectomy by means of electro-cautery. Another organism, *Fusiformis necrophorus*, was found in the tonsils after removal and thought to be the cause.[3]

Coughing is also a symptom of infestation with the cat lungworm and, overseas, with the heartworm (see chapter 6).

Acute bronchitis is accompanied by coughing, loss of appetite, fever, and breathing which is faster than normal. It may follow one of the viral infections or result from an allergy. The cat may wheeze.

Pleurisy. A later symptom of this may be a short, sharp, 'hacking' cough, but in the acute form it begins with dullness, fever, and signs of pain when slight pressure is applied to the chest walls. Breathing becomes rapid and altered in character, giving the impression that the abdominal, rather than the chest, muscles are doing all the work. After 24 to 48 hours there may be an effusion of fluid exudate into the pleural cavity. Pain is reduced, but breathing tends to be more difficult. Urgent veterinary attention is needed.

Pneumonia is a not infrequent sequel to bronchitis in a cat already ill from a viral infection. The temperature is raised, breathing is laboured, and the lips may be alternately blown out and sucked in. A short, moist cough may become very troublesome.

In broncho-pneumonia there may be a copious discharge from the nostrils during recovery, and finally a 'cast' may be expelled. (These 'casts' are formed of exudate, moulded to the inside of a bronchial tube.) Broncho-pneumonia can prove fatal within four days or so, or may persist for two or three weeks before recovery takes place.

Some outbreaks of pneumonia in catteries result from a strain of *Chlamydia psittaci*, the causal agent of psittacosis, adapted to the cat lung. Mortality can be high.[4]

In cases of chronic pneumonia the cause is sometimes a fungus, e.g. infections of the lung such as Blastomycosis, Cryptococcosis, Aspergillosis.

Tuberculosis in cats is now an uncommon disease in Britain — a situation very different from that prevailing in the 1930s, when bovine tuberculosis was rife in dairy cattle and anti-tuberculosis drugs had not yet been discovered for the treatment of human patients. Now bovine tuberculosis has been virtually eradicated from British dairy herds, and moreover nearly all milk is sold pasteurised (the exception being some milk sold by farmer-retailers). Consequently cats are far less likely to have TB, though farm cats if given raw milk straight from the cow might be unlucky enough to have it from a cow with as yet undetected TB. Another potential source of infection is knacker's meat if sold, despite the law, unsterilised. Avian TB occasionally occurs in cats, probably after catching and eating infected wild birds.

Dr A. Paredi and colleagues found between 3 per cent and 8 per cent of over 8,000 cats autopsied at the Alfort Veterinary College, France, between 1956 and 1964, to be infected with TB. This was mainly of the human type, and it is considered that most cases of TB in cats probably arise nowadays from contact with infected people.

A chronic cough, gradual loss of condition, digestive upsets, and sometimes ascites (dropsy) are among the very variable symptoms.

A persistent cough may be one symptom of **lymphosarcoma** (see Feline leukaemia, chapter 18). In a small proportion of cases it is the cough which leads the cat's owner to seek veterinary advice.

Pyothorax is a fairly common condition in the cat, and may be a sequel to pneumonia, a penetrating wound of the chest, perhaps a bite. Pus accumulates within the chest cavity. A cat with this illness is likely to rest on its brisket, be reluctant to move, show tenderness when the chest is handled, and have laboured breathing (sometimes the 'abdominal' sort mentioned under pleurisy). Cyanosis, a bluish discoloration of tongue and gums, is seen in a few cases. Treatment involves aspirating the purulent fluid and putting in an antibiotic. Unfortunately, there is only about a fifty—fifty chance of recovery.

Oedema of the lungs is seen in cases of paraquat poisoning, allergy, and exposure to smoke in burning buildings. Fluid collects and fills what are normally air spaces for the exchange of oxygen and carbon dioxide, so that the cat, in effect, 'drowns' in its own effusions. Oxygen can save life in a few cases.

Dyspnoea merely means breathing with difficulty or distress, and may follow several conditions of which coughing is one symptom, the presence of a tumour, or some forms of heart disease.

Heart disease. A persistent cough occurs with disease of the left side of the heart, and may be accompanied by dyspnoea. The cat may appear restless at night.

Disease of the right side of the heart often gives rise to ascites, sometimes to swelling of one or more limbs due to oedema. Engorgement of the veins often occurs, with enlargement of the liver. The cat becomes easily tired and may lose weight. Ultimately congestive heart failure is liable to occur.

If the above sounds alarming or depressing to the reader, please remember that a great many cats with defective heart action live to a ripe old age.

REFERENCES
1 McHowell, J. and Allan, D. *J.Comp.Path.* 74 (1964), 415
2 Lloyd-Evans, L.P. *Vet.Record* 100 (1977) 158
3 Prescott, C.W. *Austr.Vet.J.* 44 (1968), 331
4 Foggie, Angus. *Vet.Record* 100 (1977) 315

13 The Thirsty Cat

A feverish cat is likely to be a thirsty one, though thirst may be only one of the symptoms. As many cats resent and resist the insertion of a clinical thermo-meter into the rectum, I suggest that only the owners of very amenable cats should attempt temperature-taking (chapter 8). However, watch for other symptoms, and seek veterinary advice should they appear.

A thirsty cat is not, of course, necessarily feverish. For example, **Diabetes insipidus** is characterised by thirst and the passing of more urine than normal but may result from a hormone deficiency, or stress, and is treated accordingly.

Diabetes

True diabetes, *Diabetes mellitus,* is by no means rare in cats. A poor appetite and lack of energy may be noticed before the owner comes to realise that the cat is drinking more water, and perhaps passing more urine, than usual (though the latter symptom is not easy to detect with cats). After a time, loss of weight, occasional vomiting, and perhaps a cataract may be observed. Dr M. Schaer,[1] in a review of 30 cases found the most common symptoms to be depression, weakness, decreased appetite, and thirst. Loss of weight, polyuria, and vomiting were less often seen.

To say that diabetes is due to a deficiency of the hormone insulin, secreted by cells in the Islets of Langerhans in the pancreas, is still true, but medical research has in recent years revealed several ways in which the disease may arise. Viruses, such as that of mumps, may adversely affect the insulin-secreting cells; excessive doses of cortisone and similar compounds can produce diabetes, as may an insulin-antagonist circulating in the blood, or an auto-immune disease running in families. All such causes may be relevant to feline medicine, too.

From a practical point of view, the diabetic cat is unable to control the use and storage of glucose (blood sugar) derived from the carbohydrate part of the diet. Normally, when blood sugar rises above a certain level, insulin is released by the pancreas and rectifies the situation. If this fails to occur, as in diabetes, an excess of glucose in the blood (*hyperglycaemia*) persists and is removed by the kidneys and excreted in the urine.

Diagnosis depends upon urine tests and I recall a visit to a cottage to see a cat 'which was not very well'. After the owner had described such symptoms as she had been able to observe, she asked: 'Do you think the trouble could be diabetes? I have diabetes myself.' I pointed out that as diabetes was not infectious, it could only be sheer coincidence if her cat was suffering from diabetes, too. However, gentle pressure on the cat's bladder produced, without any distress, a sample of urine and, as I had a urine-testing cabinet in the car, I was able to tell her within minutes that it appeared that she was right!

Treatment of diabetes in the cat is usually successful; and cats are surprisingly tolerant of daily insulin injections. Where, however, the owner does not want to give these, insulin — or other drugs — in tablet form may be tried.

Other Causes of Thirst

Nephritis (inflammation of the kidneys) is usually accompanied by thirst and sometimes by vomiting. Old cats are not uncommonly sufferers from chronic nephritis. In order to eliminate waste products from a diminished area of functioning kidney, they need to drink more water than they used to. This, in turn, means more urine, and it may be advisable to provide two litter trays instead of one for night use.

Pyometra, a condition of chronic metritis in which pus accumulates within the uterus, also gives rise to thirst and sometimes vomiting. There is a most unpleasant discharge from time to time, in the 'open' type, but the owner may not notice this.

Thirst is evident in **feline infectious enteritis** (Panleukopaenia), but often while the cat crouches over a saucer of water it seems unable to lap.

Shock, the condition of low blood pressure which follows a serious injury, scald, or haemorrhage, is accompanied by thirst.

Intense thirst is one sign of **phosphorus poisoning**.

REFERENCES

1 Schaer, M. *J.Amer.Anim. Hosp.Assoc.* 3 (1977), 23

14 The Vomiting Cat

Vomiting is a complex act involving a contraction not merely of the stomach muscles and a dilation of the oesophagus, but also contraction of the abdominal mucles, the diaphragm, and muscles of the chest. Before vomiting occurs there is usually a profuse secretion of watery saliva, which serves as a lubricant for the passage of material from stomach to mouth.

A cat about to vomit may appear uneasy and sometimes seek a secluded place; but cats, like dogs, often vomit with the minimum of fuss, and may deliberately induce the act by eating grass. Repeated vomiting, however, can prove exhausting.

Sometimes all that is vomited is a little yellowish froth; in most instances the last meal, or a part of it, is returned.

Regurgitation rather than vomiting is a better term to apply to the ejection of partly digested food by the nursing queen, shortly before her kittens are weaned. This is a natural means of providing them with some semi-solid food, and should cause no alarm to her owner. Nor should the regurgitation of a mass of fur. This is a routine procedure among wild cats which thereby rid themselves not only of their own swallowed fur but also of indigestible material from their prey.

These two physiological instances apart, vomiting is of more significance in the cat than in the dog, especially as cats are normally fastidious over what they eat. However, a hungry cat is perforce a scavenger unless it 'lunches out' in a second household. Stray cats are reduced to scavenging in towns, and greedy or pathologically hungry cats turn scavengers.

Particularly at times of dustmen's strikes, when piles of rotting refuse collect in the streets, and the material becomes additionally infected by rats, mice, or seagulls, cats may fall victims to enteric infections — and foreign bodies, too, sometimes.

Highly seasoned table scraps may upset some cats; and a few are allergic to a certain food. This may give rise to vomiting. So, it seems, may stress.

Vomiting may occur in a cat which has come indoors after eating a toad; while retching and profuse salivation if the toad has merely been picked up by the cat (see chapter 10).

Occasionally a kitten or adult cat will vomit one or more parasitic worms. This does not necessarily indicate a heavy infestation, but it should prompt the owner to dose the animal with an anthelmintic prescribed by a veterinary surgeon.

Gastritis does not appear to be at all common in cats, except where the mucous membrane lining the stomach is inflamed at the same time as that of the intestine. For example, vomiting may occur in a case of Salmonella 'food poisoning'.

Do cats have gastric ulcers? The answer is yes, but only very rarely, and then often in association with a fungal infection in a debilitated cat.

Far more common is vomiting due to irritation caused by a fur ball or other foreign body (see chapter 15 for case histories).

Naturally, vomiting often gives rise to the question: 'Has my cat been poisoned?' In only a small proportion of cases does the answer turn out to be 'Yes' (see chapter 10).

What is called projectile vomiting, in which the stomach contents are ejected for a greater distance than usual, is a symptom of **pyloric stenosis**. This is a constriction of the pylorus, the muscular valve which controls the exit of food from the stomach into the duodenum. It is far from being a common disorder, but may occur both in kittens (in which there may be a congenital defect) and also in adult cats. It can sometimes be relieved by an operation, should this prove necessary. Projectile vomiting may occur also when there is spasm of the muscle either at the entrance to the stomach or at the pylorus. Dilation of the oesophagus often accompanies the former condition. Food may be returned very soon after swallowing.

More often than not, vomiting is the result of a disorder affecting some organ other than the stomach. For example, it is a common symptom of enteritis—inflammation of the intestine. The many and diverse causes of this are outlined in chapter 15. Reference to intussusception will be found there.

Vomiting may occur because of impaction of the large intestine by a mixture of faeces and fur, or sometimes by wool or string, or merely by retained faeces.

Vomiting and diarrhoea may occur when a cat is being transported in a basket or cage, as a result of stress or fear. In ships and aircraft, vomiting may be due not only to stress, and the noise and vibration, but also to the effect of the motion on the balancing mechanism of the ear.

Finally, do not be alarmed if your cat vomits a little froth once or twice but otherwise seems well. Repeated vomiting, however, with or without other symptoms, does indicate the need for professional aid — and that urgently.

15 Digestive System Disorders

The cat's mouth, like the face, offers a valuable guide to the animal's state of health. One looks at the gums — are they a normal pink, or pale, or tinged faintly with yellow? Is there a strong odour from the mouth? Is the tongue free from ulcers? Is the roof of the mouth congested, with engorged blood vessels attracting a longer look at the hard palate? Are the teeth free from tartar? These are some of the clues looked for in the course of the detective work which goes into the making of every diagnosis. Veterinary patients cannot talk!

Gums and Teeth

Pale gums suggest anaemia, including the specific disease **feline infectious anaemia.** Extreme pallor is seen in cases of **haemorrhage**, shock; a yellowish tinge indicates **jaundice.**

Gingivitis, or inflammation of the gums, has many causes. One of them is the accumulation of tartar referred to above, and its encroachment on to the gums. This condition is accompanied by infection and usually a foul odour. If unchecked, shrinkage of the gums is likely to occur; and later the underlying

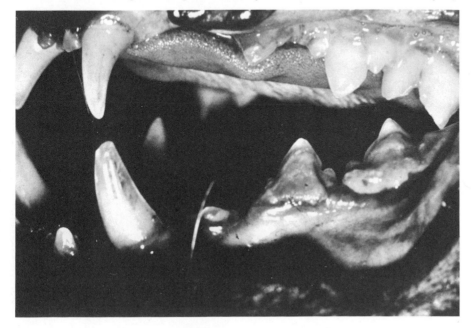

Fig 44
A deposit of tartar on the teeth, with gum inflammation.

bone may be affected. As the gums recede from the teeth, fresh sites are formed for food particles to lodge in, for bacteria, and for even more tartar. Loosening of the teeth then follows, and the general health of the cat is impaired.

There is absolutely no need for this. If the elderly or middle-aged cat is taken for a health check once a year, the teeth can be scaled and tartar removed before it has had time to build up into concretions covering and masking the teeth.

Loose teeth cause pain, and difficulty in eating. Signs of toothache may include pawing at the mouth, rubbing the face along the ground, dribbling, and miaowing. Removal of a loose tooth can have a dramatic effect on the liveliness of a cat; while removal of a large deposit of tartar can give almost 'a new lease of life' as cat-owners often say.

Sometimes the area of gum around a tooth root is very inflamed. This may indicate infection and the need for extraction — also called for when pus from an infected root has reached the skin surface via a fistula, as mentioned in chapter 3. Another tooth trouble:

Case history 1. A middle-aged cat was brought to my surgery on account of offensive breath, dribbling, and what the owner referred to as 'one bad tooth'. On examination it was found that all teeth were tartar-free and healthy-looking except one canine, at the base of which was a mass of something surrounded by an area of inflamed gum. Hairs from the cat's coat had become wrapped around the tooth and impregnated with decaying food particles and pressed down into the gum. Removal of the mass and cleaning the area in

Fig 45
An *epulis,* or tumour of the gum, subsequently successfully removed under general anaesthesia.

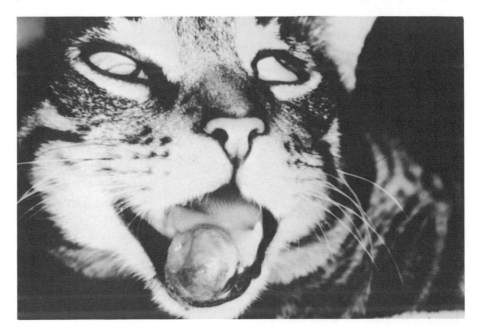

good time saved that tooth.

A more common type of foreign body is a piece of bone, wedged between the teeth, or one of those flat, almost square pieces of cartilage from ray fish (skate).

The gum may be affected by a non-malignant **tumour**, called an *epulis,* which often has a smooth, pink, rounded surface. Such a growth is not always easy to remove; and if it remains small and does not interfere with eating, removal may not be necessary. A large one is described below.

Case history 2. A 9-month-old cat had a hemispherical growth 2 cm across and ulcerated where a groove had been formed in it by the upper right canine tooth. The prognosis given for surgery was a very cautious one, but fortunately 'it shelled out easily like a pea', instead of being difficult to separate from surrounding tissue. There was no recurrence.[1]

The Tongue

A cyst, known as a **ranula,** may develop below the tongue which it pushes to one side, interfering with eating. This is a simple retention cyst due to blockage of the duct of a salivary gland, sometimes by a grass seed. Although not a serious disorder, it needs treatment in order to reduce discomfort and restore normal eating ability.

Inflammation of the tongue (**glossitis**) may be the result of unhealthy teeth or of a viral infection. Either may produce ulcers. Glossitis may be caused also by some corrosive substance which the cat has licked or by a vitamin deficiency. A kitten's tongue may become impaled on one of its own teeth, causing temporary frenzy; or a needle or other foreign body may penetrate the tongue. An inflamed tongue will make eating painful and may cause dribbling of saliva from the mouth.

The Pharynx

Inflammation of this, **pharyngitis,** may make swallowing painful, cause a cough, and be associated with a viral infection. Foreign bodies may also lodge here, concealed from view, and their detection and removal usually necessitate an anaesthetic. A piece of cotton, still attached, may help one to find a needle. Sometimes, however, this passes on to the oesophagus and beyond, or it may make a track to the body's surface.

Case history 3. 'One expects the odd scratch from a cat,' said my client; 'but yesterday I scratched myself on her. I can't understand it. There seems to be a sharp point sticking out of her skin somewhere.' There was. Protrusion had reached only a millimetre or so. Extraction of the whole needle was soon achieved. Whatever twinges of pain the cat may have felt during the needle's journey, she seemed none the worse afterwards.

The Oesophagus

Disorders here include the presence of a tumour, or of nodules formed by
Spirocerca worms causing a partial blockage, leading to regurgitation of food
in some instances.

The Stomach

Gastritis does not appear to be at all common in the cat, but may occur after
the swallowing of some irritant poison. Parasitic worms are a minor cause in
Britain. Gastric ulcers are rare. Inflammation of the stomach may be caused
by irritation from a foreign body, e.g. string from a roast joint, woollen fabric,
buttons, peach stones, etc, and the following case history shows how occasionally a fur ball may have much the same effect.

Case history 4. The owners of a semi-long-haired cat, aged five, noticed a
one-sided swelling of its abdomen, and sought veterinary advice; reporting
that the cat had been eating frequent but small meals, and had been retching
from time to time. A tumour was suspected, but an exploratory laparotomy
revealed a greatly distended stomach, from which — after gastrotomy — a
mass 15 cm x 5 cm of hair and grass was removed. The cat made an excellent
recovery, but there were several recurrences of this same trouble despite
dosing with liquid paraffin in an effort to prevent it.[2]

Distension of the stomach with gas (**tympany**) is rare in the cat, but an
emergency when it does occur since it may be followed by torsion.

Case history 5. A bilaterally enlarged abdomen alerted the owners of a two-
year-old spayed female cat, and they sought advice. The diagnosis was that
one or both of the above conditions was present and, under anaesthesia, a
stomach tube was passed, when a large volume of fluid and gas was expelled.
'In this case the cat was believed to have eaten a large number of grass-
hoppers.'[3]

Pyloric stenosis is referred to in chapter 14, but here is a case of a foreign
body lodged in the pyloric sphincter.

Case history 6. A three-year-old Persian cat had lost its appetite. On veterinary examination a hard, moveable object could be felt in the abdomen. After
radiography had confirmed its position, the object was removed through an
incision into the stomach wall, and proved to be a rubber suction cap from the
end of a child's arrow.[4]

Fig 46/47
These radiographs
show the presence of
two common foreign
bodies in the cat: a
needle, and a fishhook.

The Intestine

Diarrhoea is, of course, a symptom of **enteritis**, or inflammation of the
intestine. There are many causes. An 'error of diet' is one (see scavenging in
chapter 14). Enteritis may be due to bacterial, viral, or protozoal infections; to

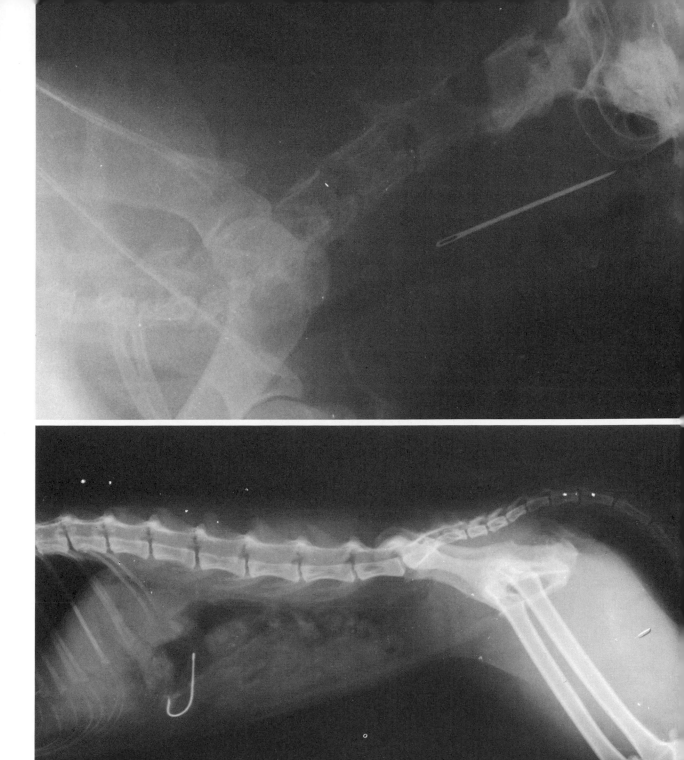

poisons; worms; allergies; and stress.

First-aid. Withhold food for a few hours, and then offer white of egg beaten up in a little milk, or milky rice, or plain boiled rice, or other light foods. Do not give cats preparations sold for human use in cases of 'travellers' diarrhoea'; but charcoal or kaolin may be suitable.

Of viral infections, **feline infectious enteritis** is not a very good example since diarrhoea is not always a symptom, especially in very acute cases. A **rotavirus** (such as causes diarrhoea in children, calves, foals, piglets) has been isolated from kittens. **Feline leukaemia** virus is an occasional cause.

Bacterial enteritis does not appear to be very common in cats, but both *E. coli* and *Salmonella* infections (common causes of 'food poisoning') have been recorded.

Protozoal infections include Toxoplasmosis and Coccidiosis; the latter not being of much importance in cats.

Dehydration is a serious consequence of diarrhoea occurring for any length of time; water and also salts being lost. In an attempt to conserve body fluids, the kidneys diminish the quantity of urine, so that there may be the added complication of waste products circulating in the blood. Dehydration is a potential cause of death, and treatment is urgently needed. Glucose-saline injections are used for this purpose.

Intussusception is a form of obstruction of the intestine — a part becomes turned in on itself. Sometimes a sausage-like swelling can be palpated. It is a very serious condition, since not only is the intestine blocked but blood vessels may become strangulated and peritonitis occur. Food is refused and great uneasiness shown. It is not uncommon in kittens. Vomiting is an important symptom. Treatment is surgical and involves withdrawing the part of the intestine which has gone inside another part.

Intussusception may be associated with prolapse of the rectum, after straining, and a sausage-shaped portion of bowel, red or bluish red, projects from the anus. There is risk of this everted part being physically damaged, so it must not be left like that, or gangrene may occur.

Case history 7. After being missing for two days, an eight-year-old neutered male returned home and was seen to have a prolapse extending for about two inches beyond the anus. Veterinary examination showed that the everted bowel was much swollen and heavily contaminated. There was no orifice, and it was obvious that manual manipulation would not succeed. Accordingly the mass was surgically removed, a laparotomy performed, and the intussusception reduced, revealing a neat hole (where the incision had been made), and this was closed. The cat made an excellent recovery.[5]

Like the stomach, a loop of intestine may sometimes become twisted (*volvulus*), with all the dangers associated with intussception. To straighten it out a laparotomy will be necessary. Occasionally a damaged portion may have to be removed, and a junction made between the healthy cut ends.

Constipation is more of a problem of detection in cats than of actual occurrence. (As previously mentioned, straining over a litter tray or in the garden may lead the cat's owner to the false conclusion that it is constipated while in reality it has a bladder near to bursting point and cannot get rid of its urine.) However, constipation can occur in cats having some other disorder, or receiving little or no roughage. It can be relieved by offering some oil out of a can of sardines, and largely prevented by including some vegetables in the diet. Regular (daily) dosing with liquid paraffin is fraught with the danger that absorption of fat-soluble vitamins may be impaired.

Impaction of the intestine by a foreign body (including a mass of fur) or of faeces and bone particles, may occur. Enemas may be needed to afford relief but are usually outside the scope of feline first-aid and may greatly distress a fully conscious cat, though not invariably so. The rectum may be empty but there may be a mass of hard faeces in the colon, perhaps owing to a diverticulum, or to other causes.

Intestinal obstruction is sometimes accompanied by the vomiting of faeces-like material. If the vomit resembles coffee-grounds it may contain some partly digested blood.

In long-haired cats which have been suffering from diarrhoea, the fur around the anus may become matted to the extent that further faeces cannot be passed. The fur must be cut away (see chapter 4).

Like the dog, the cat has two anal sacs; but unlike the dog's, these seldom become abscess sites or give trouble as a result of blocked ducts. Nor is anal fistula at all common in the cat. Here is an unusual example.

Case history 8. A three-year-old male Siamese had been off its food and listless when veterinary advice was sought. Temperature was 104°F. The main finding was swelling and excoriation of the anal region. Gland contents were pressed out, as this was assumed to be the cause, exacerbated by the cat's having rubbed the part. After antibiotic treatment, the cat was returned home. Five days later, however, the cat was back. This time a fistula was found below the tail. As a foreign body was suspected, a radiograph was taken, and this revealed a canine tooth. This was removed, the fistula treated to promote healing and ensure its closure, and all was well thereafter. Evidently the Siamese had been attacked by another, victorious cat.[6]

The Pancreas

Diarrhoea may result not only from the causes mentioned under enteritis, but also from chronic disease of the pancreas when there may be a deficiency of its protein- and fat-digesting enzymes. Symptoms often include a ravenous appetite, and the passing of malodorous fatty faeces, usually pale in colour. Treatment involves maintaining the cat on preparations of these enzymes. If the cat is amenable to this, recovery can be expected in many cases.

The Liver

Diarrhoea may occur also in some diseases of the liver. Acute **hepatitis**, or inflammation of the liver, can be produced by poisons, bacteria and their toxins, and by viruses. The liver is a common site for abscess formation, and its tissues may suffer damage from the migration of parasites; e.g. worm larvae, toxoplasms and, overseas, liver flukes. The 'liver/kidney syndrome' is discussed in chapter 16.

Symptoms of hepatitis include fever, signs of pain when pressure is applied to the abdomen, loss of appetite, a disinclination to move about, and either diarrhoea or constipation.

Subacute or chronic hepatitis may give rise to a gradual loss of condition, a staring coat, capricious appetite, jaundice and, sometimes, ascites (dropsy).

Jaundice is also seen in obstruction of the bile duct, in poisoning, in tropical and other diseases involving destruction of red blood cells, and in some cases of tuberculosis.

The liver is subject to fatty and other forms of degeneration, including **cirrhosis** — in which many of the liver cells are replaced by fibrous tissue — when jaundice and ascites may be seen.

REFERENCES
1 Schneck, *Vet.Record* 97 (1975), 181
2 Worwood, L.E. and Jones, R.M. *Vet.Record* 104 (1979), 222
3 McCamley, R.N. *Vet.Record* 102 (1978), 504
4 Mundell, J.D.C. and Gard, P.D.R. *Vet.Record* 103 (1978), 248
5 Neill, R.H. and Scott, Andrew. *Vet.Record* 104 (1979), 328
6 Rendane, V.T. and Nelson, A.R. *Feline Practice* 6 (1976), 8

16 Urinary System Disorders

Nephritis

In one survey, conducted by Dr J.M. Hamilton M.R.C.V.S., some form of **nephritis** (inflammation of the kidneys) was present in a little over 5 per cent of the cats autopsied; but this figure rose to over 23 per cent when only cats nine years old and above were considered.

Your veterinary surgeon may speak of **nephrosis**, or of the **nephrotic syndrome.** This may be a stage in nephritis, and involves damage to the tiny tubes which filter off waste products from the bloodstream. Such damage may result in protein being excreted in the urine, to the detriment of protein levels in the blood.

Nephritis may involve the *glomeruli* (small knots of blood vessels about the size of a grain of sand, from which excretion of fluid out of the blood into the tubules takes place); while chronic interstitial nephritis affects mainly structural or supporting cells in the kidneys; and pyelonephritis involves mainly that part of the kidney called the *pelvis*, where urine collects before passing into the ureter on the way to the bladder.

There are other more technical subdivisions of nephritis, classified according to microscopic findings, but in general the symptoms which the cat-owner may notice are: a reduced appetite, a tendency to drink more water, a loss of glossiness affecting the coat, and dullness or dejection. Loss of weight may occur, and occasional vomiting. While the cat becomes thinner, there may be enlargement of the abdomen ('pot belly') due to an accumulation of fluid (*ascites*).

With chronic nephritis, the appetite may not be impaired, and the other symptoms mentioned above may not be present except to a limited extent, other than thirst which remains.

Treatment of acute nephritis includes the use of antibiotics, perhaps of a urinary antiseptic also. It is usually possible to aid recovery, but the condition is apt to become chronic in the elderly cat. The diet needs changing to reduce the protein content a little. Consult your veterinary surgeon. Vitamins B and C are useful.

A cat with chronic nephritis often lives to old age — not in the pink of health, of course, because the area of functioning kidney will have been reduced, and there may perhaps be relapses, but seemingly able to enjoy life still.

Kidney failure can be a terminal illness if it leads to **uraemia** — a condition in which waste products that should have been excreted remain circulating in the bloodstream. The cat becomes very weak, vomits, and the tongue is likely to be ulcerated. This may give rise to a foul odour and salivation. There may be an odour of urine emanating from the whole cat, which is now in a critical condition and, despite intensive care, likely to die. Whether treatment or immediate euthanasia is indicated is a matter for discussion between client and veterinarian.

Liver-kidney syndrome is an illness with similarities to leptospirosis in the dog. Indeed, leptospiral infection does occur in the cat, and was found in 5.6 per cent of 233 cats autopsied by Dr J.M. Hamilton, but at the time of writing veterinary pathologists maintain that these corkscrew-shaped organisms do not produce disease in the cat. 'Liver-kidney' syndrome, since the cause is at present unknown or in doubt, is therefore a provisional name only. It affects cats mainly between two and eight years old. The animal becomes dull, not much interested in food although thirsty, and vomits.

On veterinary examination, the patient is usually found to have a slightly raised temperature and, sometimes, the yellow tinge of jaundice is evident when the mucous membrane lining the mouth is examined. In other cases jaundice does not appear for another day or two.

Treatment with penicillin, etc., may help restore the cat to health within a week or two; but in a proportion of cases there are relapses; or the jaundice becomes more marked and persists — when the cat is likely to become very thin and may die. Fortunately, this is one of the less common feline illnesses.

Hydronephrosis is a condition, far from common, in which the capsule of the kidney, or even the kidney itself, becomes distended with urine and much enlarged. It may result from obstruction of the ureter by a tumour, calculus ('stone'), or an inflammatory condition; or it may have a congenital origin.

Case history 1. Abdominal palpation of a cryptorchid cat brought to a veterinary surgery for removal of the abdominal testicle revealed the presence of a smooth, firm mass. This was found on laparotomy to be the enlarged right kidney, from which 160 ml of urine was aspirated before nephrectomy was performed, and the missing testicle found and also removed. The cat made an excellent recovery.[1]

(Of course, nephrectomy would inevitably prove fatal if carried out on one of those rare female cats having only one uterine horn and one kidney!)

Enlargement of a kidney may also result from haemorrhage into its capsule due to crushing of the organ in a road accident. Rest, and treatment to counteract shock, are indicated; and many cats then recover in about three weeks time, the blood being absorbed.[2]

Cancer of the kidney may occur during the course of Feline leukaemia.

Cystitis

Inflammation of the urinary bladder is a common condition in cats and often the result of an infection. In the female this is likely to be an ascending one, from the vagina via the urethra; while in the male a descending infection is more common, spreading from the kidneys via the ureters to the bladder.

Some cases of cystitis may be so mild as not to produce symptoms recognisable by the cat's owner; but in more severe cases the frequent passing of small quantities of urine, sometimes accompanied by straining, may attract attention; though the owner may think that the cat is constipated. In acute cases, pain may cause the cat to be restless and even to utter a cry. Professional treatment is needed.

'Feline Urological Syndrome' (FUS)

Both cystitis and osbtruction of the urethra may have one feature in common: the formation of sand-like material, composed of varying proportions of crystalline and organic matter. The crystals are usually struvite (ammonium magnesium phosphate hexahydrate). As there has been uncertainty as to how and why such deposits are formed (*urolithiasis*), the name 'feline urological syndrome' or 'FUS' appeared in scientific papers, and may be used in conversation by your own veterinary surgeon.

In a Danish survey of 345 cases of FUS occurring between 1965 and 1970, 190 of the cats had urethral obstruction and 155 had cystitis. Both conditions were more common in cats between four and six years old.

Urethral Obstruction

In cats, the sand-like material referred to above is more common than large individual deposits, but these calculi or 'stones' do sometimes occur.

Case history 2. A 4¼-year-old neutered tom cat had been passing blood in its urine, and it was this which prompted the owner to seek veterinary advice. Treatment brought some improvement but the blood was still being passed, so radiography was suggested. This revealed the presence of what proved to be, on its removal, a grey-white disc-shaped 'stone' 18 mm across and 3 mm thick. Recovery from the cystotomy operation was uneventful.[3]

Pain or difficulty in passing urine, or inability to pass any at all, is always an emergency. There is the danger of rupture of the bladder, with release of its contents into the abdominal cavity. If that happens, death from shock and peritonitis become almost inevitable. The pain which can lead to shock, is a reason in itself for veterinary treatment.

The aim of this is obviously to remove whatever is causing the obstruction. The urethra may be blocked by a particle or two of the sand-like material mentioned above, or a plug formed of this and organic matter, or even a grass seed. However removal is more easily said than done, since the cat's penis is so small, and the urethra necessarily even smaller in diameter. Sometimes one can, by gentle manipulation of the end of the penis, free the obstruction; but in other cases this proves impossible. Use of a catheter is less practicable in a cat than in a dog, since the instrument has to be so fine. Sometimes the bladder has to be emptied by aspiration of urine, or by cystotomy. Neither is free from risk.

Unfortunately, FUS is apt to recur in perhaps some 15 to 20 per cent of cats, if not more. Some veterinarians favour the addition of a little common salt to the cat's diet, in order to induce the drinking of extra water, which has the effect of diluting the urine; but your own adviser should be consulted about this.

Claims have been made for at least two calculus-inhibiting agents. Another line of treatment has been a surgical one — various intricate operations have been devised for by-passing the penis. But if the cause of FUS, as many now believe, is a virus (calicivirus or perhaps a herpes virus), a vaccine might one day become of use as a preventative.

Probably several different but interacting factors are at work in causing FUS. The numerous types of bacteria occurring in the cat's urinary system are regarded as no more than secondary invaders in FUS cases.

REFERENCES

1 Rex, M.A. *New Zealand Vet.Jl* 14 (1966), 94

2 Joshua, Jean O. *The Clinical Aspects of Some Diseases of Cats* (Heinemann, 1965)

3 Davidson, Scott. *Feline Practice* 5 (1975), 45

17 Fits, Ataxia, Paralysis

Fits

As we all know, a 'fit' is merely another name for a convulsive seizure usually accompanied by a few seconds' loss of consciousness. Epilepsy is an example. However, the word 'fit' is also applied to hysteria-like conditions in which a cat may rush about, knocking things over. A fit often leaves an animal temporarily dazed and weak. (Fits have to be differentiated from fainting, heart attacks).

Epilepsy, common in the dog, appears to be relatively rare in the cat. A chronic nervous disorder arising from brain damage, it is usually an inherited condition. The fit may occur when a cat is lying down asleep, and take the form of 'galloping' movements.

So-called secondary epilepsy may be the result of a head injury, and may occur whenever scar tissue is formed in the brain.

Without recourse to the specialist's electro-encephalogram, it is virtually impossible to differentiate 'epileptiform' convulsions from those of true epilepsy. Where necessary, drugs can be given to ameliorate attacks, or even suppress the fits altogether; drugs are not, however, the complete answer to fits, and at best should be used sparingly.

Teething and worms may account for some fits in kittens, but to a far less extent than in puppies.

Convulsions are one symptom of the effects of many different poisons; for example, organochlorine insecticides such as dieldrin, DDT, BHC; strychnine; ethylene glycol ('anti-freeze'); metaldehyde slug tablets.

A few weeks after the birth of her kittens, a queen may have convulsions as a result of **eclampsia** (see chapter 20).

Convulsions are seen during the course of several infections, especially those which can cause encephalitis or meningitis; e.g. toxoplasmosis, feline infectious peritonitis, rabies. Bumping into furniture as though blind is sometimes seen in encephalitis.

Aggressiveness is seen not only with rabies but also with benzoic acid poisoning, and some cases of organochlorine poisoning.

Ataxia

Ataxia, or a staggering gait, may arise from an upset of the balancing mechanism by streptomycin, an antibiotic which not all cats can tolerate. It occurs also in ethylene glycol poisoning, feline infectious peritonitis, and may

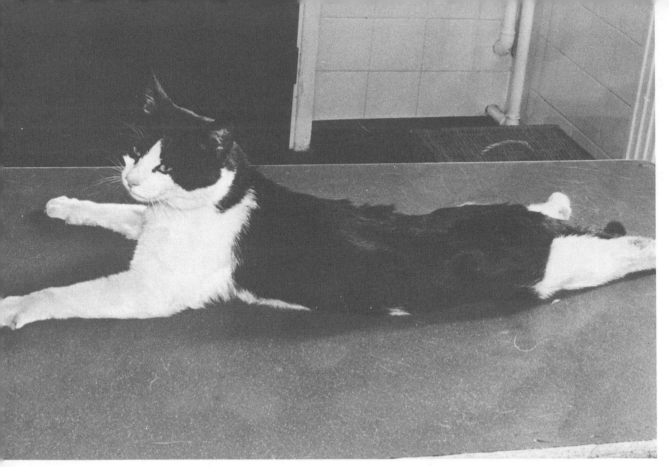

Fig 48
Paralysis of the hind
legs following a road
accident.

precede the onset of eclampsia or paralysis.

A tilting of the head may result from disease of the ear's balancing mechanism, from a tumour, or occasionally from toxoplasmosis.

A circling movement may indicate the presence of a *meningioma*, 'the most common central nervous system tumour of cats'. In a survey of 36 cases in cats 10 years old or more, Dr Lawrence Nafe noted that 10 cats circled; 11 showed drowsiness, loss of appetite, and decreased activity; and five had 'seizures', two with twitching of the facial muscles. Seven were blind.[1]

Paralysis

This may be temporary or permanent. When muscular power is merely weakened without being lost altogether, the term *paresis* is used.

Causes of paralysis are numerous and include a brain haemorrhage, thrombosis, pressure on a nerve by a tumour, pressure on the spinal cord by protrusion of an intervertebral disc, nerve injuries, poisoning, and infections.

One example of poisoning not already mentioned is **Chastek paralysis**, caused by the eating raw of certain fish whose tissues contain thiaminase, an enzyme which destroys thiamin. A staggering gait and convulsions also result from this cause. Treatment consists mainly in the administration of the B vitamins.

PARAPLEGIA

Paralysis of both hind-legs is known as paraplegia. There is complete loss of limb functions, together with incontinence as a rule. One cause is fracture of the spine following a fall from a height or, more commonly, a road accident. Blows and kicks are other possible causes. Euthanasia is the only humane course, but first a diagnosis is important, since some other cases of paraplegia may recover; for example, where there is no fracture of the spine but inflammation of the spinal cord.

Thrombosis of the femoral arteries may cause the sudden onset of paraplegia. A complete absence of pulse in these arteries is an aid to diagnosis. Euthanasia is indicated.

Between each vertebra of the spine there is a disc which has a soft, pulpy centre and fibrous or gristly outer ring. The disc acts as a shock-absorber and also supports the spinal cord at the gaps between the bones. Partial or complete rupture of the disc may occur, thereby exerting pressure on the spinal cord. The condition (which is entirely different from the human 'slipped disc') causes pain, weakness (paresis) or paraplegia, but it is relatively rare in the cat as compared with certain breeds of dog. Natural recovery may take place within a fortnight, but the outlook becomes progressively less hopeful as time goes on.

HEMIPLEGIA

Paralysis limited to one side of the body may be the result of cerebral thrombosis, haemorrhage, or embolism — plugging of an artery in the brain. The affected cat may fall over (always to the same side), or move in a circle. A tilting of the head and nystagmus (a jerky involuntary movement of the eyeball) have also been recorded. Fortunately, extremely few cat owners will ever encounter these conditions.

OTHER FORMS OF PARALYSIS

Following injury to the facial nerve, facial paralysis may occur and give a lop-sided appearance to the cat's face.

Radial paralysis is not uncommon in the cat; and may result from fracture of the first rib — the broken ends of the bone lacerating or pressing upon the radial nerve. The fore-limb is held in the position assumed at the beginning of a stride, but the toe cannot be brought forward, since nerve impulses are no longer reaching the muscles which extend the part. The elbow 'drops' and there is knuckling at the carpus. Natural recovery does occur in some instances, usually after many weeks.

AN OVERSEAS FORM

Quadriplegia (paralysis of all four legs) may result from the bite of a single tick of certain species, e.g. *Ixodes holocyclus* and *Dermacentor variabilis,* in Australia, the USA, and other parts of the world.

Eating of flesh from the Toadfish (Puffer Fish) is another cause of paralysis.

Case history. A two-year-old cat had vomited 'after exposure' to Toadfish, and was paralysed. The pulse rate was 200 per minute. Veterinary treatment succeeded in reducing this to 120 per minute, and the cat slowly improved over the next three hours. On the following day there was severe ataxia, especially of the hind-legs, which distressed the cat. A sedative was accordingly given. Full recovery occurred within a couple of days.

Dr R.B. Atwell and Dr G.B. Stutchbury, of the Department of Veterinary Medicine, University of Queensland, who treated the cat, commented that a differential diagnosis involved ruling out both tick bite paralysis and a bite by the Brown Snake.[2]

REFERENCE
1 Nafe, L.A. *J.Amer.Vet.Med.Assoc.* 174 (1979), 1224
2 Atwell, R.B. and Stutchbury, G.B. *Austr.Vet.Jl* 54 (1978), 308

18 Less Common Infections

Those described in this chapter vary from the fairly common to the rare; the latter being included for the sake of those owners whose cats are affected. Even so, the list is not complete.

FELINE INFECTIOUS ANAEMIA

It is hard to say just how common or uncommon this is, since many infected cats show no symptoms until stress or a second infection converts the subclinical anaemia into overt illness. An example of this was given in the case history at the end of chapter 2.

The cause is a single-celled parasite found in the bloodstream, and known either as *Eperythrozoon felis* or *Haemobartonella felis*. Symptoms include loss of appetite, fever, dullness, loss of weight, weakness, and sometimes slight jaundice. The cat may become very ill, and a few die; with others, relapses are common before eventual recovery.

Treatment includes the use of organic iron compounds and, in severe cases, even blood transfusion, in addition to a drug to kill the parasites. Flea control is important, since the flea is believed to be an important means of spread of the infection. During nursing and convalescence, chilling and stress must be avoided.

Diagnosis is difficult to confirm, because the parasites may not be present in the first drops of blood taken for testing.

Case history 1. A 5-month-old Burmese-cross neutered male was weak and pale about the gums, and on veterinary examination the liver and spleen were found to be enlarged. Examination under the microscope of stained blood smears confirmed the presence of infectious anaemia, and the cat was treated with a suitable antibiotic and a B_{12} vitamin preparation. Recovery followed, and 30 days later blood examination showed no trace of the parasites.[1]

FELINE LEUKAEMIA

This is a disease of major importance in the cat, and is caused by a virus discovered by Professor W.H.F. Jarrett, University of Glasgow, in 1964 or thereabouts. This virus gives rise to forms of cancer: **lymphosarcoma**, involving several organs including the thymus gland; and **leukaemia**. The virus may infect the bone marrow cells, causing anaemia, and the kidneys.

Feline leukaemia virus is readily transmitted from one cat to another, and

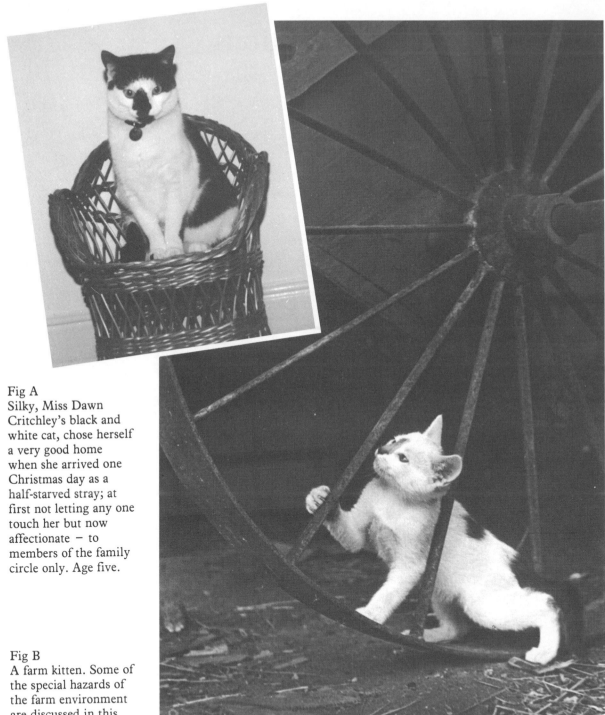

Fig A
Silky, Miss Dawn
Critchley's black and
white cat, chose herself
a very good home
when she arrived one
Christmas day as a
half-starved stray; at
first not letting any one
touch her but now
affectionate − to
members of the family
circle only. Age five.

Fig B
A farm kitten. Some of
the special hazards of
the farm environment
are discussed in this
book.

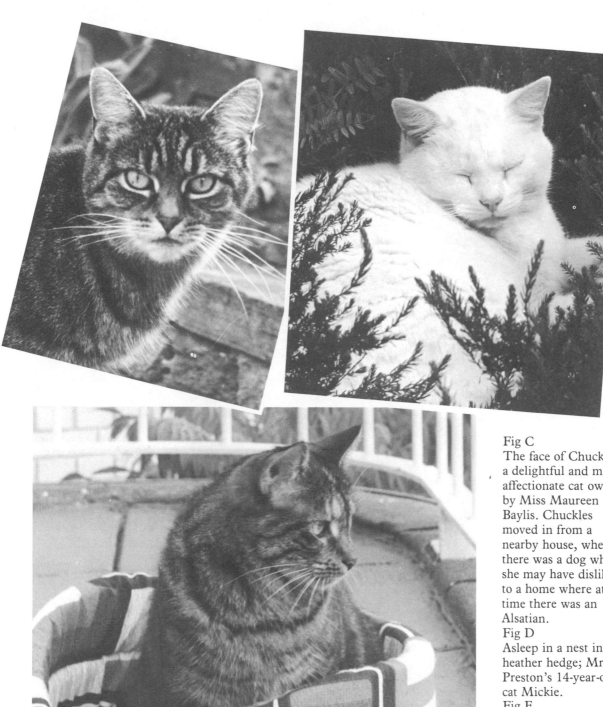

Fig C
The face of Chuckles, a delightful and most affectionate cat owned by Miss Maureen Baylis. Chuckles moved in from a nearby house, where there was a dog which she may have disliked, to a home where at the time there was an Alsatian.

Fig D
Asleep in a nest in a heather hedge; Mrs M. Preston's 14-year-old cat Mickie.

Fig E
A picture of alertness. The face of Mr and Mrs J.C. Scriven's delightful cat Frisky.

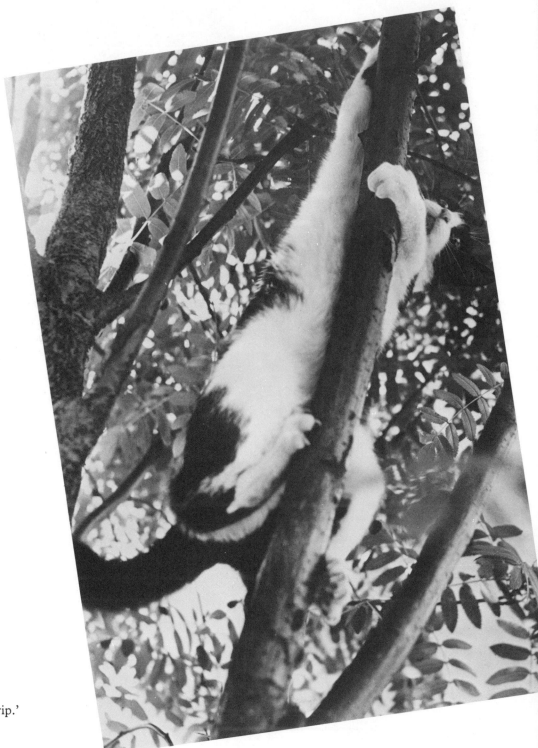

Fig F
'I'm losing my grip.'
Fig G
'Fluid motion'.

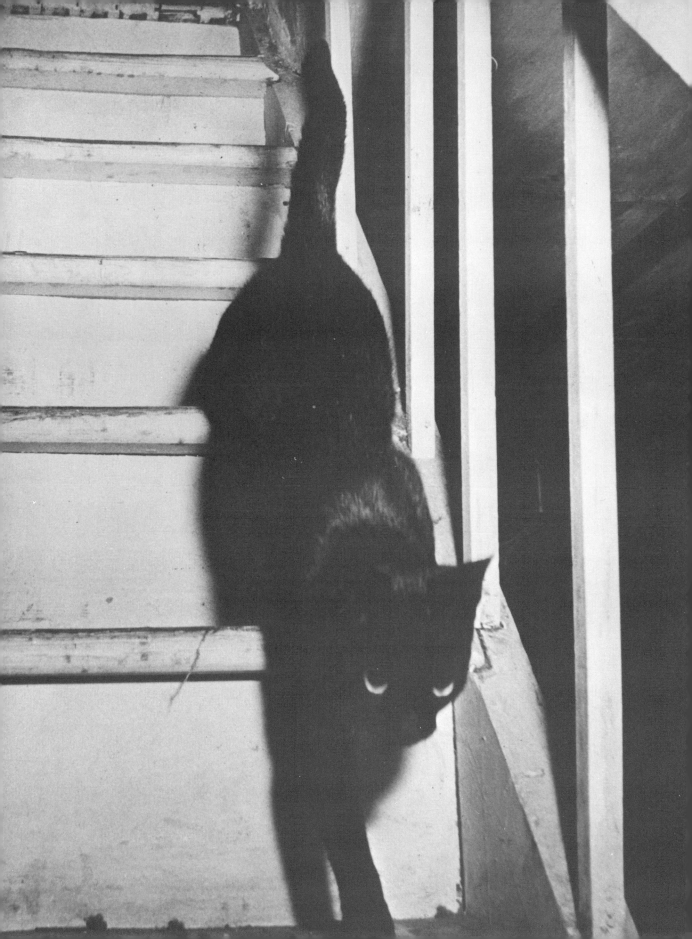

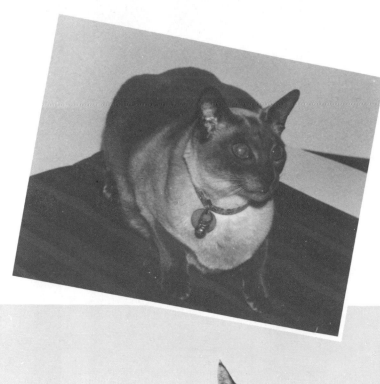

Fig H
Mr and Mrs Gordon's
Siamese, Brighton.
Fig I
A Devon Rex
photographed by Marc
Henrie.

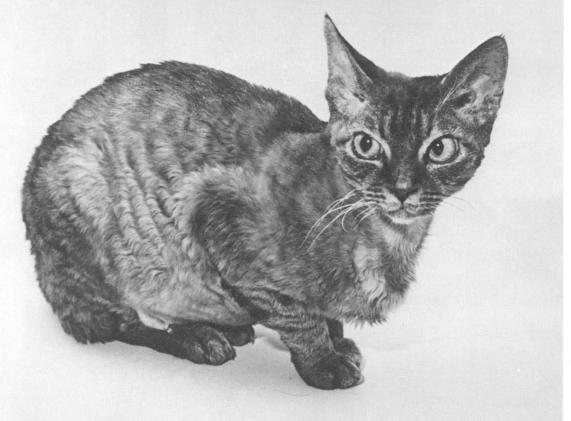

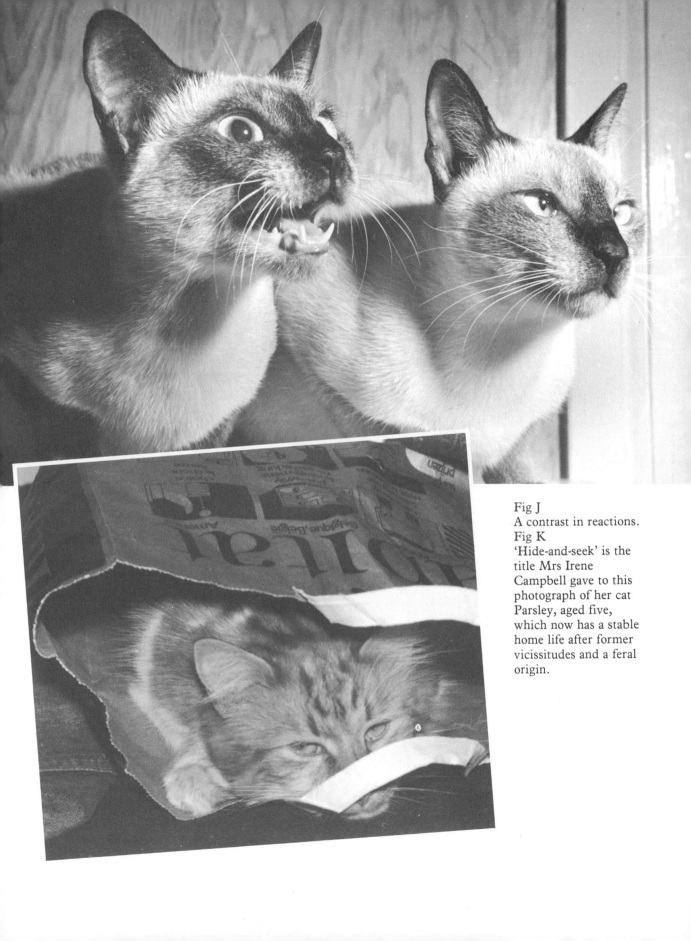

Fig J
A contrast in reactions.
Fig K
'Hide-and-seek' is the title Mrs Irene Campbell gave to this photograph of her cat Parsley, aged five, which now has a stable home life after former vicissitudes and a feral origin.

Fig L
A portrait by Walter
Chandoha.
Fig M
Sparring.
Fig N
Cat and dog;
confidence.

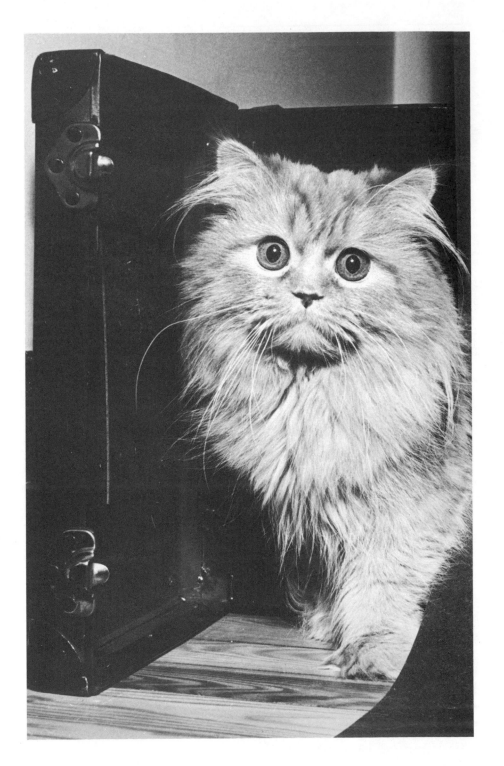

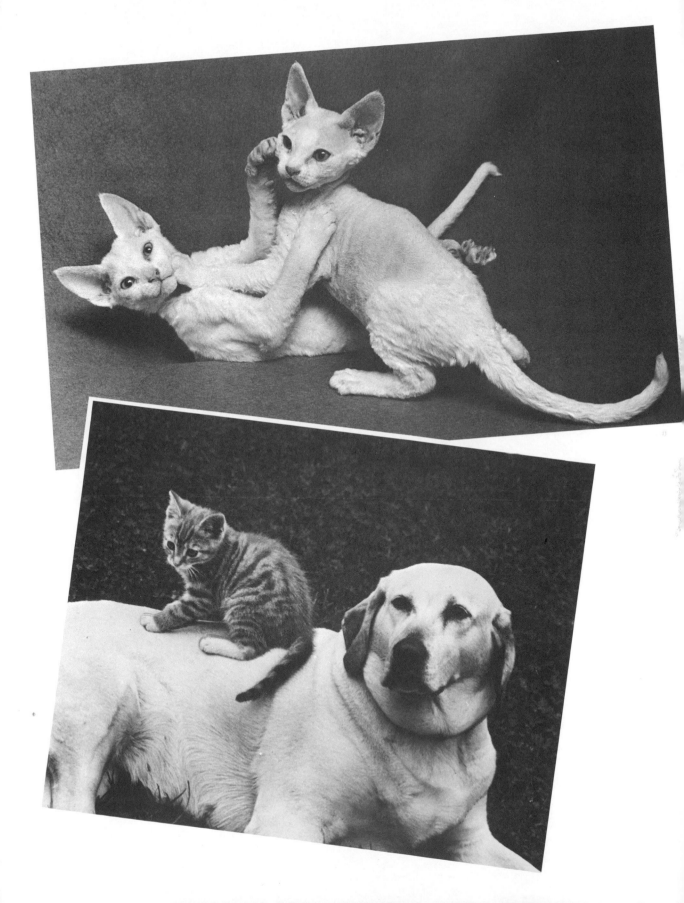

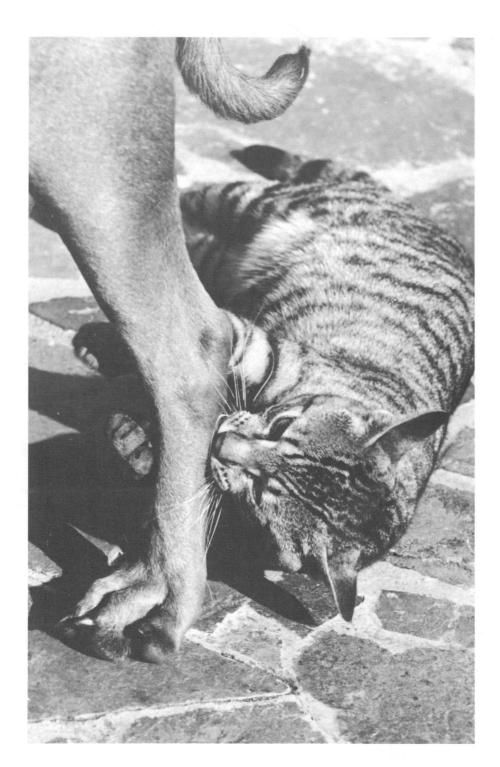

Fig O
Cat and dog; taking a
liberty.
Fig P
Cat and dog;
confrontation.

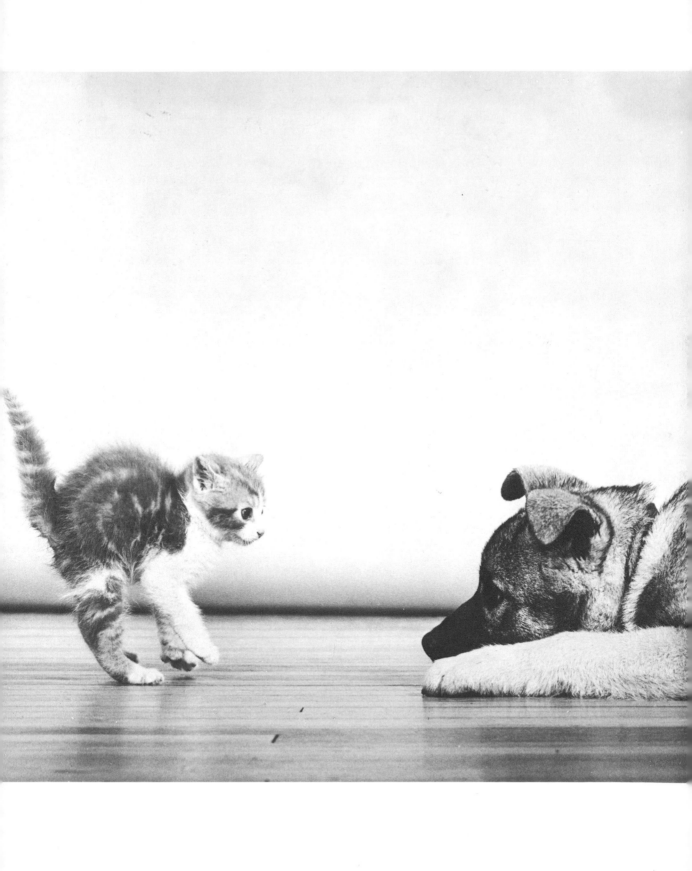

this fact is obviously worrying for the owners of catteries. When the virus is present in the blood, excretion of virus can take place via the saliva, urine and, in a lactating queen, the milk.

The infection may remain dormant for a long period. Some cats experimentally inoculated with the virus did not become ill until four years later. Fortunately, many cats are able to overcome the infection.

When symptoms do appear they are usually either (1) a gradual loss of condition, with poor appetite and an absence of liveliness, together with anaemia; or (2) laboured breathing, due to the accumulation of fluid within the chest; sometimes a persistent cough, and frequent vomiting. A fatal outcome must, unfortunately, always be expected.

Prevention may be possible in the future, but no commercial vaccine is available at the time of writing. Meanwhile, a 'test-and-remove' programme can be carried out in catteries, in which the virus is now regarded as an important cause of infertility, with abortions, stillbirths, and foetal resorption.

FELINE INFECTIOUS PERITONITIS (FIP)

The existence of this as a separate specific disease was first recognised in America. Its occurrence in Britain has been known only since the 1960s. Affecting cats mainly under five years old, FIP often occurs in association with feline leukaemia, which reduces the cat's resistance so that a symptomless FIP infection becomes an overt illness. The symptoms include fever, loss of appetite and of weight. In the so-called wet form, **ascites** (dropsy) occurs; and fluid may also be present in the chest, when breathing becomes laboured and there may be a cough. There is also a 'dry' form — much harder to diagnose — which may involve liver, kidneys, eyes, and brain. Dr Charles Povey has stated that 'anaemia is seen in 40 per cent of cases, and jaundice in 20 per cent'.[2]

Caused by a virus, this disease is usually fatal.

TOXOPLASMOSIS

This is a common *infection* rather than a common *illness*, since many cats become infected (as can be demonstrated by blood tests), show no symptoms at all, or only very mild ones, and develop a subsequent immunity. This, however, may break down under conditions of stress or of a new infection of another kind.

Toxoplasmosis is caused by a single-celled parasite, *Toxoplasma gondii*, similar in many respects to those causing coccidiosis in birds and mammals. Cat faeces may contain the parasites in one form, and cat's prey in another.

Symptoms are extremely variable, according to which organs are affected.

Young cats may become acutely ill with broncho-pneumonia. Vomiting, diarrhoea, jaundice, and inflammation of the iris are other symptoms, only one or two of these occurring in any one cat. If the brain becomes involved, there may be a staggering gait or circling movements. The acute illness is easily mistaken for feline viral enteritis. Diagnosis is dependent on laboratory methods. In older cats, toxoplasmosis may take a chronic form with intermittent fever, and it is a possible cause of abortion in the queen.

TUBERCULOSIS

A brief reference to this contagious disease was made in chapter 12, in which it was emphasised that TB is now an uncommon illness in cats in Britain. Many cases which do occur are examples of person-to-cat infections; but the avian and bovine strains of *Mycobacterium tuberculosis* still pose a threat. Catching and eating infected prey is a possible source of infection.

The disease is usually a slowly progressive one; the cat losing condition over a period of weeks or months. Appetite may be capricious. Symptoms vary greatly. There may be an accumulation of fluid in the abdomen or enlargement of the lymph nodes. Occasionally vomiting and diarrhoea occur. A deep-seated tubercular abscess may discharge pus on to the surface of the skin; and sometimes ulcerating 'lumps' form there. Liver involvement may give rise to jaundice; brain involvement to nervous symptoms. TB may flare up after a time in an acute form, with pleurisy or pneumonia. On public health grounds the disease in cats is never treated.

PSEUDOTUBERCULOSIS

Also known as **Yersiniosis,** this disease is rarely diagnosed in Britain, but in the Lyons area of France it accounts for 80 per cent of feline jaundice, Dr. H.H.Mallaret, of the Pasteur Institute, has stated. He mentioned other areas of France where the infection is rare or apparently non-existent.[3]

Cats may become infected through their prey: either birds or rodents. Non-hunting cats are unlikely to have the disease. Apart from the jaundice mentioned above, symptoms of the acute form include loss of appetite, rapid emaciation, intense thirst, and diarrhoea alternating with constipation. In a chronic form, loss of condition, a dull coat, and a tendency to crouch in a corner are seen. Pseudotuberculosis is usually fatal, and diagnosis is difficult during life.

TETANUS

This is rare in the cat. As to symptoms, the limbs show a rigidity, the tail may be held over the back, the third eyelids drawn partly across the eyes, and there may be a bow-like curvature of the spine. An exaggerated response to touch, light, or noise may provoke convulsions. (See chapter 8 for a case history of a cat which made a perfect recovery.)

ANTHRAX

In temperate climates this disease is very rare in the cat, and likely to occur only after the eating of meat originating from a farm animal dead from (unsuspected) anthrax, or of unsterilised bonemeal sold as a garden fertiliser. It is usually an extremely acute illness, and there may not be time for symptoms (of high fever, rapid prostration, and sometimes the passing of blood in liquid faeces) to be observed by the owner.

Case history 1. A four-year-old Siamese seemed normal at 7.30 a.m. but was dead at 2.30 p.m. A blood smear from the cat did not provide a 'convincing' diagnosis, but another blood smear from the same owner's monkey, which had also died suddenly, was positive for the anthrax bacillus. Both animals had eaten knacker's meat.[4]

AUJESZKY'S DISEASE

Also known as **pseudo-rabies**, this disease is caused by a virus. In Britain the disease is rare in all but farm cats, though since rats are not uncommonly infected, any cat could theoretically become ill after eating such prey. In Hungary, where the disease was first recognised, feeding uncooked lung and oesophagus from pigs has accounted for many cases. The effect of the virus is to cause a burning or itching sensation so intense that self-mutilation may occur. Other symptoms are dejection, loss of appetite, and restlessness, salivation; sometimes miaowing, excitement, and waving the tail horizontally from side to side. The disease in cats is virtually always fatal, and unfortunately there is no effective treatment.

Case history 2. On an East Anglian farm, where housed cattle shared a common air space with pigs, four calves died from Aujeszky's Disease, although the pigs had shown no symptoms other than loss of appetite. A farm cat died twelve hours after showing profuse salivation and dejection.

REFERENCES
1 Collins, J.D. and Neumann, H.J. *Irish Vet.Jl* 22 (1968), 88
2 Povey, C. *Vet.Record* 98 (1976), 23
3 Mallaret, H.H. *Réc.Méd.Vét.* 141 (1965), 1079
4 Cripps, J.H. and Young, R.C. *Vet.Record* 72 (1960) 1054

19 The Neutering of Cats

Reasons for Neutering

It may seem cynical to position in this book a chapter on neutering before one on breeding; but, with a household pet cat — from the owner's point of view, and often the cat's welfare, too — neutering is usually essential sooner or later, whether the animal be male or female.

An owner may at first find the idea of neutering repugnant, but when litter after litter of kittens have to be found homes, opinion is likely to change. The late Frank Manolson D.V.M. referred[1] to his doctor's wife, who was firmly against spaying but, after her cat had produced 120 kittens — and she had run out of friends, patients, and others who might offer a home to a kitten — finally agreed to the operation being performed.

Few owners go to such lengths before deciding to have their cats spayed, and few could hope to find homes for a quarter as many kittens. It is unwise to press a kitten on someone reluctant to accept it, for all too easily it can then become a stray, underfed and having to fend not only for itself but for the many kittens it will inevitably produce, each competing for diminishing food resources once it is weaned.

There is also the noise factor to take into account. A Siamese in oestrus, by her 'calling' can annoy neighbours, especially in a block of flats; and the noise may get on the owner's nerves, too.

It may reasonably be asked: Is there no equivalent of the 'Pill' for contraceptive use in cats? There is, but spaying is far preferable, for the following reasons. First, the owner may forget to dose the cat at the right time; secondly, some feline contraceptive preparations have had to be withdrawn by the manufacturers because of serious side-effects, so that it is best to discuss the matter with your own veterinary surgeon in the light of what is available at the time of consultation, should you still be interested.

Tom Cats

The reasons for neutering tom cats are equally cogent. While an entire male can be very affectionate, his owner inevitably takes second place during the breeding season. By the end of the latter, the cat may have become thin and gaunt. Sexual prowess is achieved at the cost of many fights with other cats, so that the animal is likely to return home on many occasions with a torn ear or an abscess following a bite, in need of veterinary treatment and of attention by the owner. The cat may have been missing for days.

The strong and unpleasant odour of a male cat's urine is a most important reason for castration, since the odour can permeate the whole house. It is true that tom cats usually confine their spraying of urine to objects outside the home, for purposes of territory demarcation and to let females know of their presence; but at times of stress even a normally well-behaved tom may spray indoors. This may occur, for example, after the introduction of a second or third cat into the home, or after a move to a new house. Aggressiveness may be a problem, too, as well as prolonged absences from home. Most catteries will not board unneutered males.

Veterinary experience is that few entire males reach the age of 11 years, since abscesses and accidents account for many earlier deaths. Castrated toms and spayed females tend to live longer.

CASTRATION

This is usually carried out when the kitten is about four months old. In the United Kingdom, castration of a cat without the use of an anaesthetic is illegal. Food and drink should not be given for few hours before the operation.

After the operation the kitten will continue to squat to urinate and will not normally spray as it grows up. The stimulus to roam the neighbourhood in search of females will never develop, and involvement in fights will be minimal. Only a very few castrated kittens become dull and lacking in character afterwards.

Owners of full-grown cats sometimes request castration in view of 'objectionable behaviour' such as urine-spraying, mounting, fighting, and wandering away from home. A study of cats following castration showed, in the words of Dr Ian Fraser Dunbar, University of California, 'a post-operative decline in fighting, roaming, and urine-spraying in 88 per cent, 94 per cent, and 88 per cent, respectively'. Improvement — especially as regards urine-spraying — was obtained in most cases within a fortnight. However, as these figures imply, a small percentage of castrated adult cats tend to carry on much as before. 'The major effect of castration is reflected by an overall reduction in the frequency of intromission, sometimes followed by a decrease in mounting behaviour.' Nevertheless, some individuals continue to copulate for quite a long time afterwards.

Post-operative care includes a close watch for any signs of haemorrhage or infection, or excessive licking of the scrotum.

Female Cats

SPAYING

In the past, this word often referred to the surgical removal of the ovaries only, but in the spaying of cats it is usual for the uterus to be removed also; i.e. the operation is a normal ovario-hysterectomy.

Most spayings are carried out between the age of four and five months. However, some veterinary surgeons advocate that the operation be performed *after* the first oestrus or, indeed, after the first litter of kittens are born. The pros and cons of later spaying should be discussed with your own veterinary surgeon, who may refer to the better bodily development which may occur if the ovaries are removed at the later stage.

What should be avoided is the spaying of a cat some weeks' pregnant, since the operation then becomes a much more serious one. Normally, spaying is a safe and straightforward operation; the cat usually returning home on the same day, with removal of stitches between one and two weeks later.

It is important always to make an appointment, and when doing so the opportunity may be taken for the cat to have a veterinary examination. In the first place, not every cat taken to a surgery for spaying is, in fact, a female; in rare instances even a tortoiseshell cat turns out to be a male. Secondly, a preliminary health check is to be recommended; and you will be reminded not to feed the cat for some hours before the anaesthetic is due.

After spaying, the vast majority of cats retain their former liveliness and affectionate nature; it is only a *very* few that suffer what, in the human being, one would call a 'personality change', becoming dull and unresponsive. In some individuals removal of the ovaries may lead to a tendency to dermatitis, a patchy loss of fur, or obesity; but hormone implants can usually overcome such effects.

Abnormalities

Occasionally some abnormality comes to light when a cat is brought to a veterinary hospital or surgery for neutering. The male cat masquerading under the false colours of a tortoiseshell has already been mentioned under 'Spaying' above; and I have seen also the unusual ginger female brought for castration on the assumption that it was a tom. Such animals are usually but not invariably sterile.

Sometimes the external appearance of the animal is normal, but a laparotomy reveals abnormality; for example:

Case history. A one-year-old tabby brought for spaying was found to have a grossly abnormal uterus, and testicles in place of ovaries.[2]

Less uncommon is the cryptorchid, in which one or both testicles have not descended into the scrotum from the abdominal cavity. A very few cats have only one testicle and are true monorchids, but this term is often used by breeders for an animal which has one testicle in the scrotum and the other inside the abdomen. The latter condition may render a cat bad-tempered and aggressive, so it is the usual practice — after removing the normally sited testicle — to perform a laparotomy and search for the other which, if found, is likewise removed.

REFERENCES
1 Manolson, F. *My Cat's in Love* (New York: St Martin's Press; London: Macmillan, 1970)
2 Heron, Mary and Boehringer, B.T. *Feline Practice* 5 (1975), 30

20 Breeding

Few people need reminding that cats are highly prolific animals, with a breeding season which extends throughout most of the year — ending in the autumn and starting again at the beginning of January or February under British climatic conditions. Three litters of kittens per year are commonplace, four not unknown.

Oestrus

Timing of the first oestrus or 'heat' is very variable, being governed to some extent by the season of the year in which she was born, but may be expected between the ages of six and eight months. However, oestrus may occur as early as 3½ months, or occasionally be delayed until the queen is about a year old.

It is usually the cat's behaviour which attracts the owner's attention rather than bleeding or swelling of the vulva, since these two signs are so slight as to be easily missed. Usually increased affection is shown, and she rubs herself against people's legs. Rolling on the carpet, quivering, and the uttering of little cries are other signs of feline oestrus, sometimes mistaken by the owner and leading to an urgent call for veterinary help with the comment: 'My cat seems to be in agony.'

The scent of the vaginal secretions, which contain powerful pheromones, attracts the male, as will her 'calling'.

There is no feline equivalent of the human menopause, and oestrus may continue to occur in the elderly queen aged 15 or so.

The Tom Cat

In the male, puberty commonly occurs at the age of about 10 to 12 months; but here again there may be considerable variation. Some toms may reach puberty as early as six months, while others do not mate until their second spring.

The tom will indicate the boundaries of his territory by the spraying of urine. The secretion of the anal glands is also probably a factor at mating time, if not before.

The Mating Ritual

The tom circles the queen and, if not rebuffed, approaches her, uttering his mating call. If she is nervous or not yet ready for him, she makes this fact plain by flattening her ears against her head and hissing at him. He may continue to pace near her or may crouch close by, biding his time. After what may be a long wait, she announces her readiness by rubbing her face on the ground, or even against the tom; rolling, treading, perhaps answering his call.

The tom then grabs her by the neck, mounts her as she crouches, and makes rhythmic movements with both fore- and hind-paws. She moves her tail to one side and assumes a position which makes penetration possible. The latter — at which she gives a cry — ejaculation, and withdrawal may all occur within a very short space of time. Immediately after withdrawal she may lunge an attack on the tom, which has usually leapt out of the way before harm can befall him. The tom soon returns, however, and settles close to her. Both perform their toilet. Copulation is soon resumed and repeated several times.

The above is the general pattern of behaviour, of which there may be variations; but of course there will almost invariably be several competing toms. These may position themselves in a circle, with the queen in the middle. The period of courtship may last hours or even days, before the acceptance of one — the victorious cat.

Once mated by a particular tom, most queens will not subsequently take offensive action against him, but will show him affection.

Mating with a second tom may sometimes occur, in which case her kittens will obviously be of mixed parentage.

In a mating planned and supervised by a pedigree-cat breeder, things will be a little different. Pedigrees will have been discussed or studied by the respective owners; perhaps a certificate of health demanded by one party, and an assurance that the queen is not vicious by the other. A written agreement may have been entered into, and this is wise. Stud cat and visiting queen will have been taken out of their adjacent cages; sometimes it is the tom which is the visitor. The queen is not always ready for him, and recaging becomes necessary, with a fresh attempt hours later. The exact time is when the queen *is* ready — a matter of the individual's physiology and perhaps psychology, not of mathematical calculation on the part of the breeder.

Precautions to protect the tom include a non-slip floor surface and a shelf on to which he can jump to escape the queen's claws once mating is completed. A second mating is usually arranged on the following day.

Ovulation and Conception

In the cat it is copulation which stimulates ovulation. Experimentally, ovulation has been initiated in the laboratory by means of a smooth glass rod — of the same diameter as the cat's penis — inserted into the vagina, when the female utters the same cry, suggesting that the latter is one of pleasure and not pain — previously thought to be due to the rough scales on the cat's penis hurting the queen on withdrawal.

Perhaps there is a mental as well as a physical stimulus. Mrs Madeline Sheppard M.R.C.V.S. suggested in 1955 that the queen watching the battles of her suitors was thereby provided with a stimulus in addition to that of copulation with the victor. She further suggested that the failure of some mated queens to conceive on breeders' premises was absence of ovulation due to absence of this other stimulus.

Pregnancy

The average length of gestation in the cat is usually stated to be 63 days. However, some litters of kittens are born on the 56th day (or even a day or two earlier), and a few after the 66th day.

The nipples of a queen pregnant for the first time may become pink and enlarged after a fortnight or so, but otherwise she shows little change during the first three weeks of pregnancy. It is not until the fifth or sixth week that abdominal swelling becomes discernible. Her mammary glands increase in size during the last few days, and milk may be present a day or two before kittening.

As this draws near, she becomes restless. She may seek human companionship or prefer solitude in some dark corner. Nest-making efforts may be observed. It is wise to help her in this direction by providing newspaper, which she can tear up, in a box placed either in a cupboard or in some other quiet, semi-dark place. In default of such provision, she may choose the eiderdown in the best bedroom, or she may obey her instinct and seek some distant place to have her kittens in privacy. Perhaps it is the conflict between this instinct and attachment to home and owner which induces a state of near-hysteria in some individuals of the oriental breeds. It is certainly advisable to confine her to the house, for some mishap may befall her if she wanders away from home.

Vomiting may occur, sometimes panting, during or before the onset of the first stage of labour. It is during this that relaxation of the pelvic ligaments occurs, together with a widening or dilation of the genital passageway. Contractions of the muscles of the uterus bring the first kitten from the horn into the body of the uterus towards the cervix which, if it has not already done so, has to relax before birth can proceed.

Birth

The first kitten is normally born within a few minutes to half an hour after the onset of the second stage of labour, in which she can be seen straining. The process of labour appears to be pain-free apart from the emergence of the kitten's head, at which she may utter a cry.

Ten minutes to an hour may elapse between the birth of successive kittens,

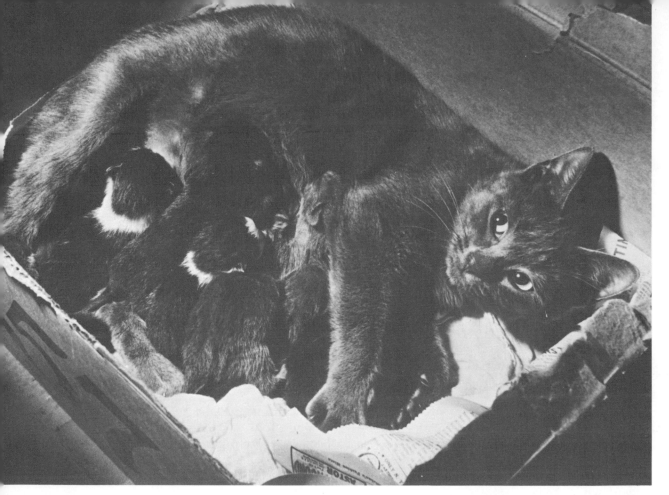

Fig 49
Mother and kittens.

but then there is a long interval of from 12 to 24 hours before the queen resumes labour and produces what might be described as the 'second instalment' of her litter.

It is seldom that human intervention is needed during feline labour, and usually the cat copes with the birth processes extremely well, attending to the umbilical cords and foetal membranes herself. Breech presentations, with the hind-legs appearing first, occur frequently and hardly ever cause problems.

DYSTOKIA

When difficulties do arise, and delivery cannot be effected by the queen herself, the word 'dystokia' is used. In a survey by Joan Humphreys of 4,077 cats over a period of 4½ years, dystokia occurred in 134, i.e. 3.3 per cent.

Dystokia is rarely the result of an oversize kitten, but is a likely occurrence in a queen which has previously suffered a fracture of her pelvis after being struck by a car. Very occasionally a malpresentation such as a sideways turning of the foetal head may render normal birth impossible, necessitating veterinary attention, and probably a Caesarean operation, since as a rule the cat's vagina is too small for correction to be achieved within that organ.

COMPLICATIONS

As indicated above, kittening is blessedly free from these as a rule, and few owners of pet cats will encounter any of the following conditions.

Uterine inertia, so common in the bitch, is rare in the cat, but the following case may be of interest.

Case history 1. Advice was sought concerning a nine-month-old queen 'on the 70th day of gestation'. On the 65th day there had been a clear vaginal discharge, but no obvious signs of labour. An injection was given, with instructions to bring the animal back in 24 hours' time if nothing happened. The following evening, a second injection was given. The first kitten, dead, was born two hours later; and three live kittens were born within a further 90 minutes. These three were successfully reared.[1]

Haemorrhage, if it occurs at all, is usually self-limiting and not fatal. **Torsion of the uterus** is very rare. The twisting may be associated with very feeble labour of the non-productive kind. Rare, too, is **prolapse of the uterus**, of which the following is an example:

Case history 2. At 4 a.m. four normal kittens had been born, but at breakfast time the queen had a Y-shaped protrusion from the vulva, and there was blood in the box with the kittens. Veterinary treatment was successful.[2]

Prolapse of the rectum, referred to in chapter 15, is an occasional sequel to straining during birth of kittens.

Ectopic pregnancy, the presence of a foetus outside the uterus, may occur in one of two ways. Probably in most cases it is the result of rupture of the uterus, such as may be caused when a heavily pregnant cat is struck by a car or is subjected to some other form of violence.

Case history 3. A pregnant ginger stray appeared and a few days later gave birth to three live kittens. After rearing these, she was spayed — when two mummified foetuses were found in the abdomen outside the uterus. An air gun pellet under the skin, and broken teeth, suggested trauma in this case, although no obvious wound of the uterus was to be seen.[3]

Ectopic pregnancy may also arise when a fertilised egg, instead of passing down one of the Fallopian tubes, towards the uterus, is released from the hind end of the tube and develops outside the uterus.

Case history 4. A mature tabby cat was brought to a veterinary surgeon for spaying, but found by him to be about to have kittens. The operation was postponed. During the night one kitten was born dead. The queen appeared unconcerned, and no signs of further labour were noted. Palpation revealed the presence of further foetuses, but with no movement and with rather a 'wooden' feel. After two hours' wait, an exploratory laparotomy was performed. Three fully formed but mummified foetuses, contained in a thin membrane, were discovered one inch from the left horn in its broad ligament, and adherent to intestine and urinary bladder. To the membrane ran a blood supply. A fourth mummified foetus was found alongside the stomach. The uterus was empty. Both sets of foetuses were removed, and an ovario-hysterectomy performed.[4]

POST-NATAL DISORDERS

Turning now to less uncommon disorders which may follow kittening, **mastitis**, involving a painful infection of a mammary gland, may occur some days afterwards. Fomentation (see p. 89) may help to reduce the pain but is unlikely to overcome the infection, for which veterinary treatment is usually necessary.

Acute **metritis** (inflammation of the uterus) is by no means rare. It may follow retention of foetal membranes, or occur if the mucous membrane lining has been damaged or become infected. Fever will make the queen dull and thirsty. She may lose interest in both kittens and food. A brownish discharge with an unpleasant odour may be noticed. She may vomit, and crouch rather than lie; or walk with the back arched and hind-legs placed further apart than normal. The illness, if severe, can prove fatal if not treated in good time. Fortunately antibiotics can be life-saving. The kittens will have to be hand fed, as she will have little or no milk and may be unwilling to nurse them; also her milk may not be good for them. Less acute cases of metritis may linger on to become chronic.

Eclampsia is rare in the cat. When it does occur, within a few weeks of kittening, hind-leg weakness, convulsions, and loss of consciousness are the symptoms to be seen. Injection of calcium borogluconate by your veterinary surgeon is urgently needed; otherwise the cat will die. (Eclampsia is also known as *lactational tetany* — a preferable name.)

Deformed Kittens

A few words on this subject may be of interest to breeders. As they well know, all breeds of livestock harbour some genetic defects. The incidence of these is usually low, but from time to time specific defects become more frequent in certain breeds. The modes of inheritance are often complex, and are outside the scope of this book; but I would like to mention two non-genetic factors which may lead to deformed kittens. The first is the use of the antibiotic griseofulvin in the treatment of an outbreak of ringworm in a cattery. It is an excellent method, but *not* suitable for pregnant queens as they are likely to produce deformed kittens following treatment.

The second factor is probably rare though not, one would think, unique.

Case history 5. After veterinary assistance, a queen gave birth to three live and three dead kittens, all showing deformities involving pelvis, hind-limbs, and tail. As the sire had a kink in his tail, the owner of the queen was very ready to assume that the cause of the kittens' deformities was genetic, and to lay the blame squarely on the sire; her cat having produced over 40 kittens in the past, all normal.

But was the cause of the deformities in fact a matter of heredity? Dr D.D. Pout, the veterinary surgeon whose client was criticising the sire, elicited the fact that the queen, during her pregnancy, had been in the habit of lying stretched out on top of a night-storage heater. He then referred to scientific papers stating that experimentally induced hyperthermia — for periods of up to one hour each day for about a week during a crucial period of gestation — produced in small mammals just such deformities as were present in this litter of kittens.[5]

Infertility

A tom may be unable to mate a queen because of some obstruction in her vagina; for example, a very tough hymen, or the presence of a polyp or other type of tumour. **Vaginitis** (inflammation of the vagina) may to some extent be obstructive but, more important, the vaginal secretions may be harmful to the sperm with a resultant failure of the queen to conceive. There may be some congenital defect of her reproductive organs which, while not preventing mating, renders her sterile. Such defects may involve vagina, uterus, Fallopian tubes, or ovaries.

The whole reproductive cycle is dependent on a delicate balance between the various hormones involved, and an excess of one or a deficiency of another may account for some cases of infertility. Such an imbalance may be temporary and self-righting or it may require treatment. A cystic ovary may result in nymphomania and infertility; so may an ovarian tumour which secretes an oestrogen hormone.

Infertility and abortion can be due to infection; for example, toxoplasmosis, feline herpes virus infection (rhinotracheitis or flu); possibly brucellosis.

Obviously, if repeated failure follows use of a particular tom, the fault may lie with him. He may be sterile, or merely temporarily infertile as a result of the stress of long confinement, or of an **orchitis** (inflammation of the testicle), or infection of some kind.

A sterile mating may lead to pseudo-pregnancy in the queen, which will exhibit nest-making tendencies and will probably come into milk.

A vasectomised tom is sometimes found useful in catteries in order to 'satisfy' queens in oestrus and reduce noise and stress.

REFERENCES
1 Nelson, M. *Vet.Record* 105 (1979), 261
2 Eggar, E.L. *Feline Practice* 8 (1978), 34
3 Humphreys, Jean *Vet.Record* 95 (1974), 353
4 McKeating, F.J. *Vet.Record* 104 (1979), 240
5 Pout, D.D. *Vet.Record* 102 (1978), 427

21 The Care of Kittens

The cat provides her kittens not only with milk but also with warmth, stimulation, cleaning, and antibodies against infection. Her presence almost certainly has some other benefit which scientists have accepted but cannot yet fully explain.

In licking her kittens, the cat imparts local stimulation to nerve endings in the skin, which in turn has an effect on their breathing, and also stimulates them to defaecate and pass urine.

The antibodies reach the kittens via the colostrum — milk secreted the first day or so after their birth. It is richer in protein and fat than her later milk; it contains vitamins A and D, and antibodies against such infections as the queen has encountered in her environment.

Initial failure of the milk supply, technically known as **agalactia**, is seldom a problem with cats. Should it occur, it can usually be overcome by administering a dose of the hormone oxytocin.

If the kittens are restless and not receiving sufficient milk, the cause could be **metritis** (see chapter 20). **Mastitis**, a painful inflammation of one or more of the mammary glands, may result in one or two kittens being in a similar plight.

The queen may neglect a kitten either because of mastitis or because of some deformity affecting the kitten; e.g. cleft palate. Kitten-killing, and even kitten-eating, is not unknown in such circumstances.

At birth, kittens weigh between 3 and 5 oz, depending on litter size, breed, etc. As a rule that weight will have been doubled by the time that they are a week or nine days old. If, with a large litter, milk supply is inadequate, it may be necessary to remove one or two kittens during the first week. Similarly, it is advisable to cull any weak or deformed kitten.

Kittens' eyes open on the 10th day after birth.

Sometimes it is necessary to trim off the sharp points of kittens' claws as they may be hurting the mother, occasionally to the extent that she is unwilling to nurse.

Supplementary feeding for the kittens should start as soon as they are four weeks old, when a little solid food should be offered — once a day to begin with. Meat, chicken, rabbit, top-quality canned cat-food are all suitable, and can be mixed or alternated. Weaning is, of course, a gradual process.

After weaning the kittens need a protein-rich diet, with four meals a day; five is not too many to begin with. One meal can consist of a dry baby food such as Farex mixed with evaporated milk or powdered milk plus water, or Munchies broken up in milk, or milky rice. Accustom the kittens to a mixed,

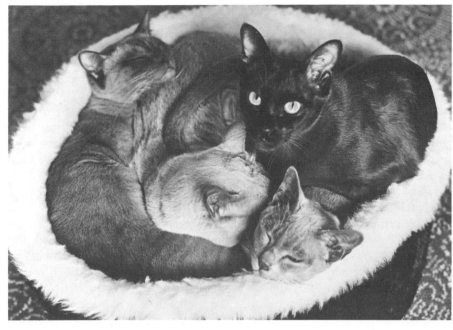

Fig 50
Watchful mother.

varied diet from early days. All the food items mentioned in chapter 2 can be introduced gradually in small amounts. A speck of Marmite can be added to the kitten's food at one meal each day. Water should be available as well as milk.

Orphan kittens, if they are to survive, need a very warm environment. A temperature of 27°C to 30°C (80° − 85°F) is recommended for the first five days; this being reduced gradually to 24°C (70°F) by the end of the fourth week. In order to provide these temperatures an incubator can be improvised from a box, warmed by hot-water bottles well wrapped so as not to burn the kittens, or by a heating pad of the electric under-blanket type, in which case there must be a waterproof layer of material between it and the kittens. The incubator box must have not only a removable lid, but also an opening, or openings, to provide light (needed after the eyes open) and ventilation.

'Place a ticking clock near the kittens', is the advice of the New York State Veterinary College, 'and separate them.' Otherwise, deprived of their mother, they are likely to suck each other's tails and navels, and 'will not get enough rest'.

Newborn kittens are best fed every two hours for a couple of days, then every three or four hours. Specially formulated kitten foods are on the market, or Lactol (intended for puppies) can be used. Cow's milk is not adequate for the rearing of orphan kittens unless supplemented as follows: for each cup of milk, add ¼ cup fresh cream (or 1 teaspoonful of butter) and ¼ egg yolk. Warm the milk, and beat in the cream and egg, adding 1 drop of cod-liver oil, advises the Pedigree Petfoods Education Centre.

Other possibilities are unsweetened evaporated milk (*not* condensed milk) or babies' full-cream powdered milk (e.g. Ostermilk) reconstituted at double the rate recommended for babies.

Kittens learn to lap by the age of three or four weeks. The saucers used should be thoroughly washed. Boiling them is the ideal.

Here are some further points about kittens, not merely orphans. **Worming** (using only an anthelmintic prescribed by your vet) can be carried out if necessary at the age of four weeks. Ask also about **vaccination** against feline infectious enteritis. Depending on local circumstances, the first of two doses is often given between six and eight weeks of age; the second dose at twelve weeks.

The kitten has 26 milk teeth. By the age of six months these have usually all been replaced by the permanent teeth.

Kitten **mortality** may be a problem in breeding premises. A single death may be due to intussusception (see chapter 15) if the kitten has been vomiting, or there may be some congenital deformity or weakness. Where numbers are dying, the cause may be an infectious disease; for example, feline infectious enteritis or feline 'flu' (see chapter 7). Hypothermia is another possible cause; likewise an incompatibility between the blood of sire and queen. See also chapter 10 for possible poisoning. Anaemia due to lice and worms is mentioned in chapter 5 and 6.

22 Cat/Man Cross Infection

'The healthy, well cared for cat presents only a minimal risk of being a reservoir for infectious disease,' commented Dr E.H. Kampelmacher, of the Netherlands Institute of Public Health, 'as compared with the great number of strays in many communities.'

Several infections can pass in both directions, that is from person to cat, and from cat to person; while others are one-way infections. In the former category, when an outbreak of illness occurs, it may be difficult to establish which introduced the infection into a household — the person or the cat. In many instances, moreover, the cat, like man, is an incidental host.

Of the **anthroponoses,** or person-to-cat infections, **mumps** provides an example. A cat may have enlarged parotid glands, and perhaps appear slightly unwell, as a result of becoming infected in a household where a child is ill with mumps.

Domestic cats have been shown to be susceptible also to some strains of **human influenza** virus, (for example the Hong Kong virus type B), so that during human influenza outbreaks some cats may become feverish or sneeze; others developing antibodies but not showing symptoms.

Of the two-way infections, **tuberculosis** is an important example. As explained in chapter 18, many cases of TB in the cat are now probably of human origin, following contact with an infected person in the same house. (Cats, like people, are susceptible to the human, bovine, and avian strains of the *Mycobacterium tuberculosis*.) There is a public health danger from a cat which has TB, and such an animal is accordingly never treated, once a diagnosis has been made.

Cats may become ill during human outbreaks of '**food poisoning**' due to Salmonella organisms, for example. It is another example of a two-way infection, since it might be introduced by a hunting cat having eaten infected prey. Equally, the source of illness in both people and cats may be contamination of hands, cook's utensils and kitchen working surfaces by uncooked poultry or 'pet's meat' originating from a knackery and not a butcher.

In the following example of **Salmonellosis**, the cat was one of two animals which passed on the infection but neither of which was its source.

Case history 1. A cat and a dog occasionally drank from a pet turtle's pool. The two-year-old daughter of the household was taken ill with severe gastro-enteritis needing hospital treatment. *Salmonella java* was isolated from the faeces of the child, the cat, the dog, and the turtle — regarded as the source of this outbreak.[1]

It should be added that some cats, like some people, may be 'carriers' of

Salmonella for a time; excreting the organisms but not showing symptoms.

Of one-way infections spread from cat to man (*zoonoses*), the most important is **rabies**, of which the cat is merely an incidental host. Chapter 23 is devoted solely to this terrible viral disease and its prevention.

Toxoplasmosis, in contrast to rabies, is primarily a feline disease in that the definitive hosts of the coccidian parasite involved are the genera *Felis* and *Lynx*.

While blood tests indicate that many cats have been exposed to this infection, it often causes (as explained in chapter 18) only mild symptoms, which may not be noticed by the owner and are followed by some degree of immunity. Undoubtedly many cat-owners, and certainly all veterinary surgeons in small animal practice, must have been exposed to infection, and have developed immunity too.

The only real danger to human health appears to be 'acute generalised toxoplasmosis, especially in persons undergoing immunosuppressive therapy', to quote the World Health Organisation; and also congenital infection which may result in abortion, stillbirth or abnormality. 'Where a woman is pregnant and serologically negative for Toxoplasma, it is recommended that any oocyst-excreting cat should be removed.[2]

Dr Kampelmacher, whom I quoted at the beginning of this chapter, commented in 1975: 'The public should be reliably informed in order to avoid the type of emotional outburst' (in the Netherlands) 'where, on the one hand recent publications have cost the lives of many cats, and on the other hand provoked serious threats to the author of an article in which he underlined the potential risk from cats to pregnant women.'[3]

Case history 2. A farm outbreak of toxoplasmosis involved birds, which are recognised as a significant reservoir of infection. Fifty chickens, reared in a building, were in the summer turned out into the farmyard, and after a fortnight deaths began to occur. Within three months only a dozen survived. The cause of death was established as toxoplasmosis, and laboratory tests also showed that antibodies to Toxoplasma were present in a mare, 23 out of 24 cows, all the farm cats, the farmer, his wife, their daughter, but not their son. The source of infection was 'probably wild birds, as various species had been found dead around the yard during the summer'.[4]

Visceral larva migrans is the invasion of human internal organs (rarely eyes) by nematode larvae which migrate, but do not normally mature, in man. Larvae of the dog roundworm *Toxocara canis* have been principally associated with human **Toxocariasis**, but other species (including *Toxocara cati*) have been recorded in a small minority of cases.

Toxocara eggs are sticky, and adhere to the animal's coat, so that a child's hands may be contaminated. Fortunately the eggs passed out of the host animal are not immediately infective if swallowed, but require a period of development in a suitable environment before becoming infective. The soil of public parks, playing fields, grass verges and gardens is commonly infected.

'Many patients with proved toxocariasis have not owned or had close contact with a dog or a cat,' the World Health Organisation has commented, but have become infected through environmental contamination as mentioned above. 'Even though eggs are unlikely to mature on an animal's coat, infective eggs from the soil may adhere to the hair so that contact with it can lead to infection.'

Ringworm is among skin diseases transmissible from cat to man (see chapter 5). The risk of human **scabies** from a cat with notoedric mange is very small, since the latter is now very rare in cats in Britain.

REFERENCES

1 Kaufman, A.E, US Public Health Service, Atlanta
2 World Health Organisation. *Parasitic Zoonoses,* Technical Report No. 637, 1979
3 Kampelmacher, E.H. *Vet.Record* 97 (1975) 104
4 Beauregard, M. *Canadian J.Comp.Med.Vet.Sci.* 292 (1965) 236

23 Rabies

An acute, infectious disease caused by a bullet-shaped virus, rabies takes its name from the Latin word for madness. 'Hydrophobia', an old name for rabies in man, is altogether inappropriate to apply to the disease in cats, in which fear of water is not a symptom.

Transmission

The commonest method of transmission of rabies virus to man and domestic animals is by the bite of a rabid animal; saliva-contaminated scratches or deep puncture wounds made by its claws providing a secondary means.

Transmission will depend entirely on the presence in the saliva of the rabies virus at the time the attack was made. This, of course, implies infection of the salivary glands.

The quantity of virus present in the saliva, and the position and severity of the wound(s) are factors which (together with the degree of susceptibility or resistance of the host) influence the development or otherwise of the disease and its incubation period.

Infection of brain and salivary glands is often but not always concurrent. If it is, as in most cases of 'furious' rabies, conditions are favourable for virus transmission; that is the animal has the urge to bite, and the bite can convey the virus.

However, infection of the salivary glands may occur *before* brain involvement resulting in symptoms. For example, foxes may secrete virus in their saliva for up to 17 days before symptoms appear. Cats' saliva could also be infective a few days before; and this represents an additional hazard for people licked by a rabid animal about the lips, nose, eyes; or for an animal licked on its nose, etc.

Once inside the body, the virus invades the nerves and, after an interval (the incubation period) reaches the brain and spinal cord, later becoming disseminated through many organs and tissues of the body. Some virus is also distributed via the bloodstream.

Since the rabies virus can produce disease in all warm-blooded animals, its victims vary from mammals to birds, from cat to camel, from tiny mouse to massive elephant. Not all animals are equally susceptible. Foxes, jackals, and wolves are extremely susceptible; cattle, cats, and rabbits are highly susceptible; dogs moderately so, according to a World Health Organisation (WHO) classification.

In Europe the fox is the main vector of rabies. Other wildlife creatures

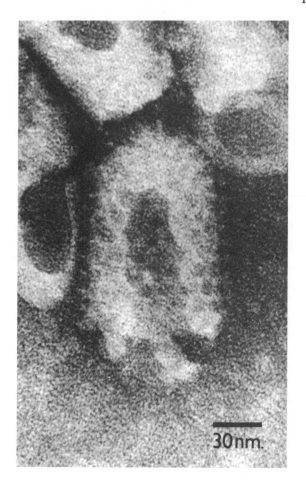

Fig 51
The bullet-shaped
virus which causes
rabies, as revealed
under the electron
microscope.

affected to a less extent are roe deer, badgers, martens, stoats, weasels, and polecats. In 1978 WHO commented: 'In areas affected by wildlife rabies, dogs and cats still represent the most important transmitters of the virus to man — forming the link between wildlife and human beings.'

While in many countries rabid dogs remain the principal rabies hazard for man, requiring his preventive treatment, in a few European countries dog-bites necessitate this to a lesser extent than cat-bites. For example, in 1969 more people needed post-exposure anti-rabies treatment following cat-bites than dog-bites in Belgium, Luxembourg, Denmark, and Switzerland.

In the last-named country over the past ten years, rabies was found in over 6,000 foxes, 285 cats, 262 head of cattle, 179 sheep, and 38 dogs (35 of which had not been vaccinated as required under Swiss law). Three people died of rabies in 1977, following contact with a cow, a cat, and a dog, respectively. In some cantons cats have to be kept on a lead while out-of-doors, otherwise they are liable to be shot as strays.

In France in 1972 confirmed cases of rabies included 36 in cats (compared with 29 in dogs); and a surprisingly high cat:dog ratio as regards rabies incidence is seen in the following table abridged from one published in the *Royal Netherlands Veterinary Association Journal*. The figures related to 1976.

Country	Dogs	Cats
West Germany*	45	58
France**	9	18
Austria	3	13
Switzerland	—	6
Belgium	—	7

(* 34 districts; ** 18 *départements*)

Symptoms

A slight fever and some loss of appetite often pass unnoticed, but then some slight change in behaviour may attract attention. A rabid cat may show extra affection. There may be a strange look about the eyes, restlessness, and a tendency to hide in dark places since the virus affects the eyes, causing some degree of photophobia.

Dr L. Andral, France's Inspector General of Veterinary Services and Director of the Rabies Research Centre, Nancy, commented at a BVA congress: 'From the outset, any change in the usual behaviour of an animal, whether it be sudden aggressiveness or excessively low spirits, any difficulty in swallowing or mastication which might appear to be caused by the presence of a foreign body in the upper alimentary tract, must be regarded as possible indications of rabies.'

Vomiting is another, though not an invariable, symptom.

The 'furious' form of rabies is far more common in cats than in dogs. Indeed, it occurs in some 75 per cent of rabid cats, and Dr Andral has described it as 'an aggressive and destructive madness, accompanied by extreme excitability'. The cat may arch its back, unsheath its claws, 'foam' at the mouth, and its normal voice become altered. Cats, like human beings suffering from rabies, may show the symptom of aerophobia, the draught from a fan being sufficient to provoke convulsions.

As can be imagined, with its sharp claws and teeth, a rabid cat is a formidable and dangerous animal; the more so as it seeks to attack the face or other part of the head in many cases. Moreover, it may remain fastened to its victim, owing to its jaws being locked in spasm.

Roughly a quarter of feline rabies cases are of the 'dumb' type; that is to say, the 'furious' phase is omitted and, after the first observed change of behaviour, the 'dumb' or paralytic stage ensues. The cat may salivate,

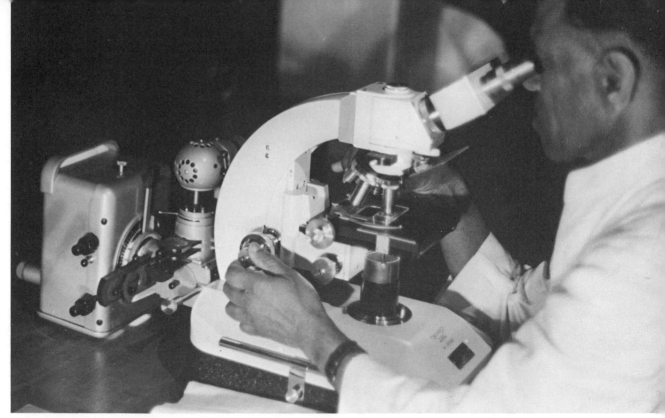

especially after it has become unable to close its mouth completely, owing to paralysis of the jaw muscles. This paralysis is gradually progressive, extending to the pharynx and larynx, so that swallowing becomes difficult and the cat dumb, and then to the limbs. Purring, however, is quite common.

Occasionally a cat is found dead with no preliminary symptoms of illness having been observed. Unless this occurs inside a quarantine cattery, rabies is unlikely to be suspected, and disposal of the body may be fraught with some danger to the person handling it.

Fig 52
Was the cat rabid? Confirmation of diagnosis being made by the immune-fluorescence test, which requires a dark-field condenser and a source of ultra-violet light.

Differential Diagnosis

Although the virus is often transmitted violently by tooth and claw, it is important to think of rabies as an insidious disease. It may occur where least expected, and the symptoms be suggestive of some entirely different feline illness.

Diagnosis during life is by no means always easy, since not all the symptoms mentioned above appear in every case. Sometimes, in fact, the illness runs a course which is far from typical. Moreover, some of the symptoms are common to other diseases; for example, feline infectious enteritis, Aujeszky's disease, tetanus. A brain tumour may bring about a change in temperament, as well as rabies. Convulsions may be a symptom of poisoning, or follow brain damage in a cat struck by a car. Salivation is profuse in a cat with a bone wedged between its teeth. Frenzy is seen in benzoic acid poisoning.

All this goes to show that a differential diagnosis is called for, and imposes a heavy responsibility on the veterinary surgeon. He has to bear rabies in mind at all times, even in a country where the disease has not been present for many years.

Vaccination

Dr Konrad Bogel, of the World Health Organisation, emphasised in 1978 that 'children are particularly at risk, and it should therefore be obligatory for all families to have their dogs and cats vaccinated when wildlife rabies spreads into their area'.

Animal vaccination has proved remarkably effective in controlling rabies in both cattle and dogs in many parts of the world, and it is very effective in cats too; but while compulsory vaccination of dogs is government policy in numerous countries, in some of them vaccination of cats is not enforced. In that situation many cat-owners fail to take advantage of feline vaccination. This fact is held to account for a reduction of only 59 per cent in the number of rabid cats in the USA between 1953 and 1971, as compared with a 96 per cent reduction in the number of rabid dogs.

Vaccination of cats against rabies involves no more than an ordinary intramuscular or subcutaneous injection of a small dose of vaccine; this dose being repeated (and this is essential) after a specified interval. An annual booster dose is recommended.

Do vaccines ever fail to protect? There are circumstances in which failure may occur; for example, if the cat happens to be already in the incubation stage, vaccination is likely to prolong this without preventing the disease. (The normal incubation period is about two to four weeks, but it can be much longer.) As with human beings, in a small percentage of animals antibody formation does not take place to the necessary extent due to some failure of the individual's bodily defence mechanisms.

While the UK remains free of rabies, British policy is *not* to vaccinate cats; but in the event of an outbreak occurring, compulsory cat vaccination would — in the danger areas — be one weapon at the disposal of the State Veterinary Service.

Smuggling of animals represents the greatest threat to the UK's present freedom (at the time of writing) from rabies. Known illegal landings of cats in 1976 totalled 45. A visitor from overseas and a British woman together brought in illegally from the Continent a dog and two cats. Any elation at having dodged Customs at Dover and saved the cost of six months' quarantine for the three animals must have been short-lived, for their smuggling activities came to light in Yorkshire and each was sent to prison for four months. And, of course, they had to pay quarantine charges after all.

Magistrates can impose fines of up to £1,000 and a Crown Court up to one year's imprisonment and/or an unlimited fine.

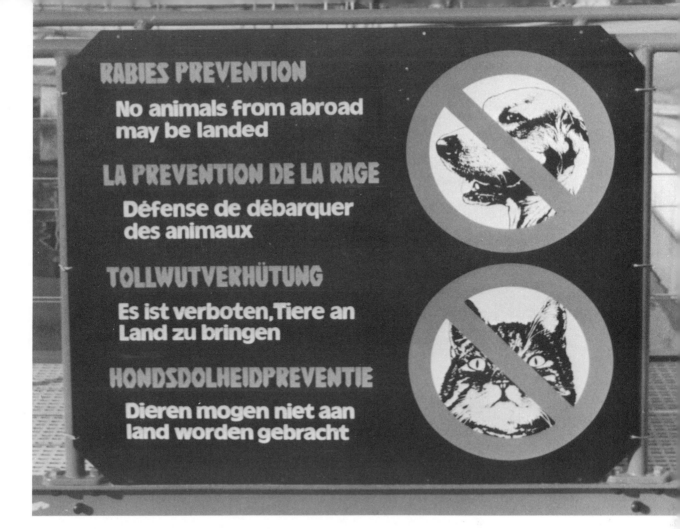

Prosecutions during 1976 totalled 125, including 34 for failure to confine animals properly on board ship or yacht.

Mr C.D. Cooke M.R.C.V.S. pointed out in a letter to the *Veterinary Record* that even if a ship's cat does not go ashore in a foreign port, local cats may come aboard to visit her. During one voyage he was presented with a queen suffering from dystokia. One bloated and decomposing kitten prevented normal delivery, and could not be removed. Ovario-hysterectomy was the obvious course, which Mr Cooke adopted as, even if the kittens had not been infected, he would not have resorted to a Caesarean operation. 'I had voyaged with puss two years earlier,' he wrote, 'and knew of her habit of coming on heat only when in port. The crew were efficient in rounding up her *inamorati* after sailing but one wondered rather, particularly after having met a rabid cat which had bitten a dozen assorted humans!' (Mr Cooke added that the ship-board surgery was uneventful, and that next morning his patient jumped into her usual daytime bed — a drawer under the chart-room table always jammed in the open position for this purpose. 'The Commodore of the line was impressed.')

Fig 53
Rabies precautions: a notice at Brighton Marina.

Importing and Exporting Cats

Many cat-owners (including experienced travellers completely familiar with passports, visas, and vaccination certificates) overlook the fact that it is illegal to take cats across many national frontiers, unless local regulations have been fulfilled. Some nations impose a total ban on cats from countries where rabies exists; others require prior vaccination and production of a certificate; or the cat may have to remain in quarantine for a specified period (four months in some countries).

Anyone intending to take a cat into the UK must obtain an import licence *in advance* from Import Licence Section, Ministry of Agriculture and Fisheries, Government Buildings, Toby Jug Site, Hook Rise South, Tolworth, Surrey, England. Arrangement for transport to approved quarantine premises, for a six-months' stay at the owner's expense, must also be confirmed in advance of the cat's arrival.

A Personal Emergency

Supposing you suspected that your cat had rabies, what should you do? First, confine the animal in a room, making sure that all windows are closed. Second, telephone the police. Third, if bitten or scratched, wash the wounds immediately with soap and water or, if available, Cetrimide. Fourth, obtain medical advice without delay.

Glossary of words not listed in the Index

aetiology	cause, study of causes
anoestrus	not in oestrus
anorexia	loss of appetite
anthelmintic	a drug used to expel parasitic worms
ascariasis	infestation with *Ascaris* worms
anuria	passing no urine
atypical	not typical
avitaminosis	a vitamin deficiency
bradycardia	slow heart action
clonic spasm	brief, spasmodic movements of a muscle
dorsal	uppermost; towards the back
dysphagia	difficulty in swallowing
dyspnoea	laboured breathing
endocarditis	inflammation of the heart's lining membrane
epistaxis	bleeding from the nose
fomites	infected objects; e.g. a cat's collar, bedding, etc.
haematemesis	the vomiting of blood
hypertension	high blood pressure
hypotension	low blood pressure
lesion	any injury or tissue abnormality
melanoma	a type of tumour, black-pigmented
metastases	secondary growths, spreading cancer
myiasis	infestation of wounds with fly maggots
neoplasm	a tumour
parietal	relating to the wall of a cavity
pica	abnormal appetite
progestogen	a drug used in suppression of oestrus and acting like the hormone progesterone
pruritus	itching
pyrexia	fever
strangury	difficulty in passing urine
subclinical	an infection not giving rise to symptoms
syndrome	a group of symptoms
tachycardia	fast heart action

tachypnoea	rapid breathing
titre	'high titres' means, in practice, that the blood serum contains high levels of antibody to a specific antigen, e.g. rabies virus
tonic spasm	continuous spasm
urolithiasis	the formation of 'stones' or sand-like deposits in the urinary bladder
ventral	undermost; towards the belly

Index